Yes!
You Can Do This!

Yes!

You Can Do This!

Charting Your Way to Health, Wealth, and Success

For
Katrina
Enjoy your journey
G Arthur Hammons

G. Arthur Hammons

arthurhammons.com

ISBN: 978-0-578-10847-6

Printed in the United States of America

Yes! You Can Do This!
is dedicated to my wife Virginia Foster
for her constant love,
encouragement and inspiration.

Contents

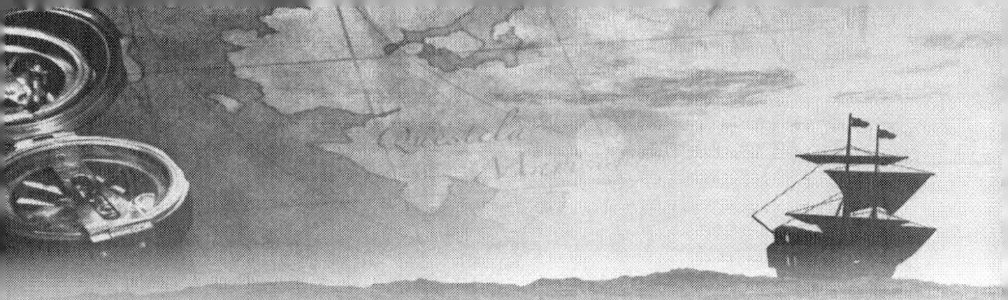

Introduction: Terra Incognita: Your Old World vs. Your New World

Conquering any difficulty always gives one a secret joy, for it means pushing back a boundary-line and adding to one's liberty.

~ Henry Frederic Amiel (1821–1881), Swiss writer

I was hanging on to the edge of the world. Salty water was pouring over me. I think I was holding on to a root or a piece of seaweed, and as I looked to each side, the water rushing past me looked like Niagara Falls. I thought—I *knew*—I was going to be swept off the edge of the earth, into the great abyss yawning under me, and die.

To my left I saw a great black sailing ship flying a pirate flag, its skull and crossbones fluttering in the ferocious wind, and its ropes and sails being flung about. A cannon rolled forward as crew members dangled from the ropes and fell into the churning sea. The ship came to the same edge I was clinging to and dipped; I could see below the waterline when the stern rose in the air, and amid the screams of the crew, the howling of the wind, and the sound of breaking masts and boards, the ship fell into the dark void below.

Something big caught my eye on my right, but, as I turned my head to see it, something enormous emerged from the water in front of me. All I could see was a huge yellow eye surrounded by scales—scales that covered the gigantic head of some kind of sea monster with fins that rose in peaks off its back. As it swam past me, it looked as long as a train. A school of strange fish and even what seemed to be a mermaid followed in its wake. By the time I focused on whatever was on my right, I realized that it was another huge ship. This one looked more like an ocean liner, and it, too, was about to experience the same fate as the pirate ship had just moments before.

Then, I saw her. I'd have known her anywhere; she was the most beautiful girl in fifth grade, and there she was: Betty Mosher, my secret love. Betty was wearing a white dress with puffy sleeves and a pink sash. With outstretched arms and desperation on her face, she called out my name, "Gary Art!" in that sweet little voice of hers. ("Gary Art" is my name in Texan.)

Her lips moved again, and she called out, "Gary Art! What is the answer?" But this time the voice wasn't hers. Now, I distinctly identified the voice of Miss Long, my fifth-grade world history teacher at Sudie L. Williams Elementary School in Dallas, Texas.

Suddenly I found myself back in my classroom. Three of the fingers on my right hand were still clutching on for dear life—to the inkwell on my desk—and my left hand gripped the top of the desk.

"Gary Art, please answer the question," Miss Long said.

The question? What question? Where were we? Where was I?

Then came that sinking feeling: *Here it comes again. I've been called on, and I don't know the answer, and my reputation for being stupid is going to get another notch in it.* The feeling rushed over me as surely as those gallons of water had moments before while I was clinging for life on the edge of the world. However, the cause of this feeling was familiar. Thanks to my many "out-of-the-classroom experiences," I had the reputation for being stupid, and whenever I was called upon, I never knew the answer.

In spite of this familiar experience of being called upon and its predictable outcome of not knowing the answer, due to a lack of paying attention, a little spark of self-defense said, *Wait, I know this.* I had always been intrigued by this place, but I never knew that it had a name. I reminded myself I had just learned the name, and, using the "peg" system my uncle had taught me, I had placed a picture of this place on a "peg" in my mind; today this process would be called remembering by association. I rushed into my retrieval system of memories to find the answer—not just for Miss Long, but also for my reputation as the stupid daydreamer who never got anything right. I knew I had just learned the answer to the question, and I truly believed I could find it. But I had to hurry; Miss Long was waiting.

I frantically started searching for that peg I had just created. The first thing I saw was Scarlett O'Hara, on her knees in the turnip patch, tears in her eyes, and her hair askew. She straightened up, and, with fists of dirt in her hands, she gestured toward the heavens and she swore something—

I had found it, or at least a part of it. I blurted, "Tara!"

Miss Long cocked her head slightly and had a "go ahead" look on her face.

Then I went searching for that second peg and conjured up a picture of my Aunt Effie May. She hated the name "Effie" and preferred to be called "May." Aunt May was my favorite aunt. Not only was she a character who always had something fun and funny to say, but she could sing, and she sounded exactly like Patsy Cline. She also looked like Patsy Cline—so much so that she was often stopped and asked if she was Patsy Cline. In response, she would adjust her sunglasses and put a finger to her lips in a "don't tell anyone" gesture. Then she'd say, "These sunglasses always make me—"

And that's when I blurted out the rest of the answer: "Incognito!" Then I repeated the answer: "Tara incognito!"

Close enough. With a look of utter bewilderment combined with praise and recognition, Miss Long said, "You're right."

Then she went on to repeat what she had said earlier: "Terra incognita is that place on ancient maps where most explorers were afraid to go to make new discoveries. They were afraid because they thought the world was flat, and they'd either fall off the edge or be killed by sea monsters."

Then she looked at me with that oddly divided expression again, as if checking to make sure that I had actually been paying attention, and still in disbelief that I correctly answered the question though I had had my familiar faraway look on my face. She must have been satisfied, so she said again, "Gary Art gave us the right answer."

For the first time in an exceedingly long time, I felt great about myself. I even thought it possible that my reputation as being "slow and stupid and out of it" might have a chance of changing. And things did get better—so much better that the sun broke through the clouds, and I could hear soft harp music and birds singing when I looked at the row of desks on my right and caught the eye of Betty Mosher, the prettiest girl in fifth grade—who gave me the biggest, brightest, most approving smile before turning her attention back to Miss Long.

I thought I had died and gone to heaven. Two near-death encounters in one day: The first one was when I just missed being eaten alive by the monster, and the second one was when I received the smile of Betty, and I survived both of them!

This experience helped me create my first formula for success. Here it is:

I was hanging on the edge of the world. Life asked me the question. I believed I could find the answer. I searched for it, and I woke up with the answer. Having the answer and giving the answer, I became a success and collected my reward.

That day, on some level, I realized that for the rest of my life, to be a success and to yield all I was hoping for, I'd have to keep coming up with answers and solutions— which I now believed were within my reach. I also knew I was the dreamer type, easily distracted and with a wild imagination. I knew I'd have to discipline these traits if I was going to be a success.

As you read and process this book, I hope you'll feel the same way I did that day—as if you're having an adventure as you enter the undiscovered possibilities that await you. I believe this area is where the discoveries, the riches, and the treasures wait to be found. You can find these undiscovered possibilities and then bring them back to your old world, to use as building materials to create a new reputation for yourself.

Manifesting results has an impact on the old you and the new you that you are creating. There might be roadblocks, challenges, sweat, and even a tear or two, but I strongly believe that accepting the invitation and meeting the challenge will be worth every bit of effort and application.

Sparking the Beginner's Mind

The idea of beginning again can be challenging. That lazy part of us says, "Well, if you don't like me the way I am, why don't you just go away?" But a new spark of possibility of what can be next says, "Yes, let's go for it." The new spark seems to know that it can light the way to new possibilities and that things the way they are now are worn out. The new spark of creativity says, "We've done it before, and we can do it again, only better. Let's go!"

A great place to start is with a beginner's mind. Creating a beginner's mind requires coming to any situation clear of all the preconceived ideas and methods that would prevent you from receiving the new experience and all it has to teach and bring out in you. One attitude that might limit your ability to absorb all the new information that awaits you is the "I already know this stuff" little voice that shares so freely from within. How many everyday things occur that are missed because we think we've seen it all, done it all, and been there for it all? How much more wonderful and adventurous could each day be if we practiced developing a sense of awe? What if you expected wonder and adventure?

Your adventure might be to learn a new skill, such as skiing or golfing. Or you might picture yourself on an African safari. Perhaps your secret ambition is to speak before an audience of thousands or appear on television before an audience of millions. If you project an aura of confidence, I believe that others around you will give you their attention and be curious. At that point, you might be able to solicit their help and give them yours, so everyone around you would reach their goals, too.

My passion for this process of going from the familiar into the unknown with the spirit of an explorer is the motivation for creating this book. I've devoted my life to teaching and living out this philosophy, and my journey has been an incredible one. On my own route to terra incognita, I had the privilege of being coached by many teachers and individuals who helped me further my understanding of how this process works. I've also encountered my share of "monsters" who I thought would eat me alive but who actually turned out to be sources of some of my best learning experiences. Likewise, I trust that I've been an inspirational teacher and example to the many people who attended the Unity church that I founded and where I served for 38 years.

In the chapters that follow, I've included many examples of what awakened individuals have done with their lives. The results others have achieved might have started with a spark of inspiration from my passion, but they brought themselves to the desired results through their own determination and the hard work they did while using many of the steps I call my map to terra incognita. Read on to discover what others have done using these principles.

As you read, perhaps you'll discover and uncover *your* next greatest journey through *your own* unknown, bring back a wealth of capabilities, and use them to expand and embellish your responsibilities, projects, and dreams.

Keep looking for those uncharted territories and new shores; you're bound to discover something new. I'll be with you every step, and our adventure will be enlightening and rewarding. Bon voyage!

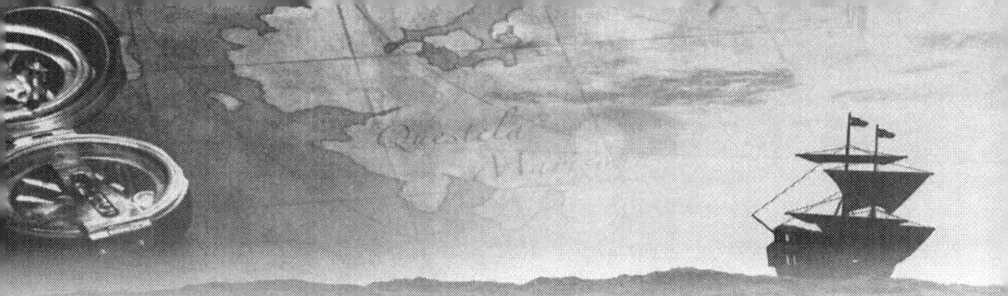

Chapter 1

Standing on the Shoulders of Giants: Other Great Discoverers

I not only use all the brains that I have, but all that I can borrow.

~ Woodrow Wilson (1856–1924),
28th president of the United States

EXPLORERS to the New World began the Age of Exploration, which history knows as the era during which explorers sailed through the barriers of fear of the unknown to new lands and made sensational discoveries that changed the perceived size and shape of the world forever. They changed everyday thinking from the concept of flat to one that had dimension. The Great Exchange was a global exchange of cultures, plants, animals, and concepts. Columbus set sail for Asia to bring back exotic spices, gold, and other goods. Instead of reaching his destination, he found a new land filled with new and exciting items; he also encountered unfamiliar cultures, and saw strange and unique animals. Europeans thought this a splendid opportunity to expand their borders, produce valuable commodities, and develop new settlements. The Spanish, Portuguese, French, and English began to mine silver and gold, grow tobacco and sugar, and build settlements for their overpopulated countries. The Great Exchange forevermore changed the landscape of life, the perceptions of people, and the world.

Your exploration into your own unknown will lead to profound discoveries as well. You can start thinking about it as your own Age of Exploration and your Great Exchange. Some of the great examples you have to follow are Christopher Columbus, Walter Raleigh, Lewis and Clark, Neil Armstrong, Balboa, Richard E. Byrd, Jacques Cousteau, Magellan, Marco Polo, Vasco da Gama, and Sir Francis Drake. There is no end to what you can discover about yourself. There is no end to what you can bring into your life from your quest. The reputation you have, with yourself and others, is what will change the most. Others will see you differently. They will have new things to say about you, and new descriptions of what you do and the way you do it. Like the explorers Hernando de Soto, Henry Hudson, and Rene Roberto de La Salle, they might even name a car after you!

> *We are like dwarfs standing (or sitting) on the shoulders of giants, and so able to see more and see farther than the ancients.*
>
> ~ Bernard of Chartres (died ca. 1130),
> Humanist philosopher

You can gain knowledge and encouragement from knowing how others overcame challenges to live successful lives. As you acquaint yourself with their stories, your awareness of how to reach your own success will be stimulated and grow. As Bernard of Chartres termed it, I call this "standing on the shoulders of giants." Rather than reinvent the process of getting to the place you want to be, you can use the techniques and styles of others to help you get there.

I, too, find inspiration and motivation as I study the success stories of others—stories filled with how they faced and overcame their challenges. (I'll also be sharing some of my personal collection of stories in later chapters.) Perhaps you'll find your favorite "giants" among them. Just a peek at the lives of some giants gives us a sense of how they took on their challenges and turned them into opportunities. I think of them often when things get tough for me. Keep in mind that these great discoverers had no guarantees that their explorations would result in success. And they didn't have any idea that what they discovered would have the impact it did. Here are some examples that come to mind when I'm in need of their inspiration:

Sir Walter Raleigh was the guy who reportedly spread his cape over a mud puddle in the path of Queen Elizabeth I. This bold but gentlemanly act earned him the right to become a member of her court and eventually one of her favorites. Likewise, his quest for discovery and adventure led him to a life where he was an explorer, writer, poet (he wrote "The Lie"), courtier, soldier, aristocrat, and spy. His desire to explore led him to establish the first English colony in the New World, to explore South Carolina, and to discover the City of Gold (El Dorado) and the Indians of Roanoke. He made many trips to the Caribbean and brought tobacco and the potato (unknown to Europeans at the time) back to Queen Elizabeth. Raleigh served in Parliament and had a secret marriage to one of Elizabeth's ladies-in-waiting, fathering three sons, two of whom survived. Later he was imprisoned in the Tower of London for treason and was accused of plotting to kill Elizabeth's successor, King James. Even with all this, his life displayed his boldness and uniqueness. He was released from prison to do exceptional tasks as a soldier and explorer for the king. His life ended, many think unfairly, when he was beheaded, and even the Beatles sang about him in their song "I'm So Tired."

I can merely imagine the history he saw during his 66 years. Imagine his being one of the favorites of the queen and going off to explore in a ship she had built just for him; his life of extravagance, love, and passion; and his being paid for his service. On the other hand, consider what he must have gone through as a prisoner in the Tower of London. I often wonder how he mustered the courage to step out into the unknown and the deep sense of accomplishment he celebrated with each success he encountered.

Another giant I admire is the Russian empress Catherine the Great. She expanded the Russian frontier, developed government administration, vigorously pursued the policy of Westernization, and gained the reputation of an enlightened leader because of her devotion to principle, and her passion for making Russia a significant country and making life better for her subjects.

Born a princess in Germany, she went to Russia at the age of 15 to meet the immature and disagreeable Grand Duke Peter, age 16. They married and had two children, but there was never any love between them. Catherine was a sensuous woman married to an insensitive man, and, although amorous interests were important to Catherine's personal life, she never let them overshadow her intellectual and political interests. She cultivated a keen interest in reading, spoke German and French, and learned to speak Russian to communicate her devotion to her subjects. Determined to be recognized as a true Russian, she adopted the country's official faith (Orthodox Christianity) and created ways to win the admiration of the people. She easily overthrew her unpopular and disliked husband and appointed herself "Catherine II, Empress of Russia" only six months after she and her husband were crowned.

As Russia's leader, Catherine proved capable and enlightened in domestic and foreign affairs; she knew the importance of creating peace within her country and with foreign powers. She was greatly influenced by the ideas of enlightenment. She belonged to a circle of 18th-century rulers who believed that a wise and benevolent ruler, acting according to the dictates of reason, could ensure the well-being of his or her subjects. She reformed the Russian legal system, expanded the country's educational facilities, and increased trade, which brought economic benefits to her people. She gave a lot of attention to the arts and science, and made St. Petersburg one of the most dazzling capital cities in the world. Her patronage of music, theater, painting, and the Academy of Science made Russia one of the major cultural centers at that time.

A piece of history that has always inspired me is the story of how doctors and scientists came to Catherine with an imported vaccine from England for the cure for *infantigo* (known as *impetigo* today), which was killing large numbers of Russian children each winter. As the physicians presented their ideas, they shared their great fear that the vaccine could be a plot from abroad to kill the children and weaken the future of the country—that it might not work and that it was some kind of poison. They suggested that they needed someone to try it out on. Showing her bravery and knowing that the need for the vaccine was imperative, Catherine promptly rolled up her sleeve and said, "Inoculate me. I'm prepared to do all I can for my subjects!" This story melts my heart, just as it melted the hearts of the Russian people hundreds of years ago.

Standing on Catherine's shoulders helps me also imagine the delight and the downsides of being born rich. I can see the responsible direction she took in life (unlike many of her wealthy peers) and how determined she was to use the gifts she had been given to benefit others. I can also imagine the dilemma and conflicted emotions she encountered being sent away to marry a difficult man she didn't love while knowing that this marriage would allow her to make changes that would create a better world.

Catherine is a great example of someone having many advantages and choosing to do all she could with what she had to work with while developing herself rather than snuggling into a comfortable lifestyle. I wasn't born with a silver spoon in my mouth—I think it was more like a Dixie cup—but, like Catherine, I think we are all born with the ability to choose. The way Catherine made the most of every situation and did it royally is an inspiration to me. By standing on her shoulders, I can see the benefits of disciplined and enlightened thought and energized actions.

I am also inspired by the accomplishments and risks others encountered that led them to great discoveries and the ability to overcome challenges. One of my favorite discoverers is the symbol of humanitarianism, the founder of the American Red Cross, and the "angel of the battlefield": Clara Barton. Although her life was filled with challenges, she was fueled with a desire to help humanity by sharing her passion for service and doing what was in her power. I trust that learning about her will give you something to recall when things get rough for you as you explore your own unknown.

Clara was the youngest of five children and was educated by her older brothers and sisters. She was so intelligent and well-read that she became a schoolteacher at age 15. Students had to pay to go to school in 1836, and Clara knew this would prevent many from getting an education. She offered to teach without salary if the school would allow students to attend for free, thus establishing the first free school in New Jersey. Enrollment went from six students to 600 students. Clara Barton is recognized for establishing free public schools because of her passion for doing the right thing for others.

From there, Clara broke another barrier: becoming the first woman to hold a government post by working in the Patent Office in Washington, DC, in 1860. I believe her quest for discovering her gifts and abilities took her to the places she needed to be, and put her in contact with the people and circumstances she needed to accomplish her calling. She clearly gathered no moss as she explored her own terra incognita, and each event in her life led her to exploration and fulfillment. Being in Washington when the Civil War began put her in the right place at the right time to pursue her passion. She served the federal troops by making appeals for provisions to be carried to the battlefields. She collected the much-needed supplies and personally distributed them. This put her on the battlefield during combat. Her mission wasn't primarily that of a nurse; instead, she became increasingly adept at passing out provisions, displaying courage and compassion as she did so. While engaged in this activity, she perceived the need to identify missing and dead soldiers. She set up the Bureau of Records and traced some 20,000 dead and missing Union soldiers and prisoners of war. This was an enormous task, and I can imagine the comfort it provided for the families of these soldiers and the achievements President Abraham Lincoln made possible as he gave Clara permission to set up the bureau.

Her humanitarian efforts reached far outside the borders of her country of birth. In her late 40s Clara went to Geneva, Switzerland, to recover from an illness. The head of the Red Cross, which was founded in that country, knew of her valiant efforts and success in helping others, and urged her to seek the United States' agreement to the Geneva Convention and to recognize the work of the Red Cross. Her efforts were interrupted by the Franco-Prussian War, but, as usual, she found a need wherever she was; she offered her services to the grand duchess of Baden and administered military hospitals. She also had the idea of putting needy women in Strasbourg to work, sewing garments for pay. Later, she went to the starving and defeated city of Paris to spearhead the distribution of much-needed food and clothing. For this, she was awarded the Iron Cross of Merit by German emperor William I. (Note the unexpected rewards that come as one follows his or her dreams, desires, and goals while at the same time being of service.)

At the age of 56, Clara Barton wrote to the founders of the Red Cross, offering to lead an American branch of the organization. She incorporated the American Red Cross, and her extraordinary efforts brought about United States ratification of the Geneva Convention. Serving as president of the American Red Cross with a passion for social service took her all over the United States, assisting victims of floods, earthquakes, fires, famine, and a tidal wave. She was invited to share her skills in Russia, Turkey, and Cuba, where she also made a difference.

Clara Barton spent the last days of her life living in the remodeled warehouse that was built for her by the developers of Glen Echo community in Maryland, just outside of Washington, DC. Her home (which is a museum today) served as a shelter, a workplace for her staff, and a storehouse for disaster supplies and Red Cross files. People in Washington knew that if they needed a place to stay or they were having other difficulties, they could go to Clara's home and she would help them. She demonstrated her giving spirit right until the end.

Clara Barton lived to be 91 and had an adventurous life filled with travel, accomplishment, recognition, and excitement, not to mention hard work and danger. I doubt that she had any idea of what lay ahead as a child, but I believe in her heart of hearts she heeded a call to go forth and discover and serve. She followed this calling, and it took her to her own terra incognita, where she made discoveries, brought them to the attention of others, and improved the quality of life for many despite huge obstacles.

I reminded myself of Clara's diligence and determination many times during the process of acquiring the necessary education and experience qualifications to serve as a minister. Remembering that her bravery and passion helped her overcome many obstacles was an inspiration to me. This is why the "angel of the battlefield" gives me plenty of inspiration as I go through my own conflicts, when things get tough for me, and as I follow what I call the calling of my heart. I trust that one of your heroes will do the same for you and that as you make a success of your life you will become someone's hero.

So, if *we* are going to go to terra incognita, let's think about what we'll discover and what we want to bring back. My experience of going to the unknown turned out to be more than I could have ever dreamed. I thought I knew what I wanted to discover, and yet what I wound up discovering was off the charts. This was because I was basing my expectations on my present charts. The same was true about what I thought I would bring back. My results from my new world discovery were not on my old world charts.

It is important to have goals, and it is imperative to put them in writing! I like to think of written goals as charts that guide our thinking with thoughts of success. In future chapters, we'll explore this further. As ideas, nudges, and urges to move forward come to you, make a note of them and translate them into a list of things you hope to discover and bring back. Keep an open mind to the possibilities of better things to come. Of utmost importance as our journey begins is to have a sense of anticipation and of being ready, and don't let your history hold you back. Think of building a future that will become your new history. Think of it as your new job!

Even after reading the inspiring tales of these great adventurers, you might still be asking, "How do I let go of the past and move into the future?" I suggest that you come to a place that's both a starting and an ending place—a place where you turn the page and are ready to begin again. In this place, you decide that you're ready to release and let go of what held you back and are ready to make the most of your present and your future. As you reflect on the events of your past, you'll recognize successes and failures, gains and losses. You'll find that each event taught you something, and made you wiser and more capable of stepping into your own unknown, to make greater discoveries than anything you encountered in the past. Knowing this, you will be in the perfect frame of mind to release the past in gratitude and take that first step forward.

In contemplating the adventure that awaits you, you're sure to experience feelings of excitement and apprehension. But remember: You can choose to be in touch with what motivates you. Are you motivated by your spirit of exploration and accomplishment? Are you motivated by the belief that you can make discoveries and claim new territory that will upgrade and influence your future? Are you motivated by the belief that your determination will empower you to meet every situation with confidence and strength? With these motivators in mind (and the memories of giants who have gone before you and probably felt as small at their beginnings as you might feel), you can release your concerns about letting go and stepping into your future.

Your self-talk at this point might sound something like this: "I'm ready to release my view of my past, and I'm ready to create a new image of myself for my future. I'm ready to stand tall right where I am. I appreciate the present moment, and I'm excited about what awaits me on this wonder-filled journey on which I'm about to embark. I'm also thankful for the past and the richness it has given me, which backs me up and has prepared me to be here on the edge of something new. I feel perfectly balanced between the blessings of the past and the promise of the future. This is my moment of power and action. I am ready!"

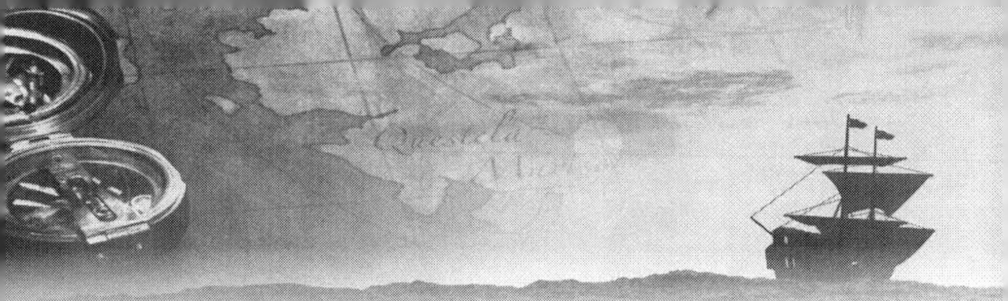

Chapter 2

Know the Power of Your Thoughts

Man's mind stretched to a new idea never goes back to its original dimensions.

~ Oliver Wendell Holmes, Jr. (1841–1935),
Supreme Court justice

HERE'S how you get what you want in life: Change your thinking.

Knowing that you have the power to change your thinking is a very powerful concept. Taking charge of your thoughts and reforming your thinking will open new vistas of possibilities and success for you. You may ask: "How is it possible for me to change my thinking?" It is possible because you have the power to discipline, organize, and reorganize what you are thinking. Best of all, you have the power to change your thinking so that it serves you and helps you to reach your goals. In this chapter, you will learn that you can change your thinking and reform your thoughts. You'll also learn the first step: knowing that every feeling begins with a thought.

I think, therefore I am.

~ René Descartes (1596–1650),
philosopher and mathematician

Did you hear the joke about Descartes? You may remember his famous quote: "I think, therefore I am." He stopped thinking for a couple of seconds, and then he died!

Some people insist that feelings come before thoughts. But the truth is that to have a feeling, you must first have a thought. Thoughts produce feelings. This step is one of the first things to learn about your thinking process. Often we have what I call runaway feelings. These feelings are so overflowing with passion they cause us to react. They often get us into trouble. We wind up saying, "If I had only stopped to think, I would not have spoken or acted the way I did." You might already have guessed that thoughts produce feelings and that feelings are a result of thinking. If this idea is new to you, then now is the time to absorb this valuable and helpful information. Your future success (and your success with others) depends on this fact.

This next bit of information might sound a bit harsh, but bear with me. The way your life is now began with an idea. The way things are now is a direct result of your thinking. The good news is that you can change your thinking and the way your life is now will change.

Perhaps this example will be helpful. Early in our marriage I completed a stained-glass window. As I proudly showed it to my wife, Virginia, she asked, "How will it be framed to hang in a window?" I mentioned that I would get some molding and make a frame for it. Virginia mentioned that that would take time that might be better invested in more creativity. Then she asked me about how long I had been doing stained glass and what my first memories about being an artist were. I explained that my first artistic expression was coloring with crayons. When she asked me to tell her about my crayons, I told her about a shoe box filled with bits and pieces of crayons of every size and color. She asked, "Did you ever have a new box of crayons?" I reminded her that, while our home was a loving one, luxuries like a new box of crayons were not a possibility. We made do with what we had by putting things together rather than going out and buying something new. Virginia then said, "Rather than repeat the pattern you grew up with, what if you go to a custom frame shop and have a really nice frame built that would be as nice as the beautiful creation you have made? You surely can afford it."

This conversation stopped me in my tracks, as I flashed back on my childhood and that shoe box of crayons. I realized that my present style of creating reflected an idea I was still attached to. This idea sounded something like "You have to make do with what you have or create it yourself; there isn't enough to go out and get what you want." I realized this idea that was given to me; it was not an original idea of my own. I realized the way my creative life was at that time began with this idea. I realized my thinking was causing me to make do with bits and pieces rather than go out and have what I wanted. The way things were began with an idea. The way things were was a direct result of my thinking. Knowing the power of my thoughts, I decided to change my thinking, which produced change in my life.

Realizing my stained glass was deserving of a proper frame, I went to a frame store and purchased one that set off my efforts. This change in thinking from "There isn't enough, so make do with what there is" spilled over into every area of my life and expressed itself as improvement that could be seen and enjoyed.

Let's go back to the idea that the way your life is now began with an idea and the way things are now is a direct result of your thinking. Much like the thoughts I had been thinking that were holding me back from having what I wanted, perhaps the thoughts that you have now were instilled in you while you were growing up. Possibly your way of thinking came because you grew up with people who got their thoughts from the same thought pool as everyone else in their surroundings. Maybe things would be better for you now if early in life you had had a coach who guided your thought processes. Yes, it is possible that you could be better off today in several areas of your life if you had known long ago that your thoughts would shape your here and now.

On the other hand, remember that your successes and accomplishments reflect a state of your life that began with an idea. You can see that this thinking principle goes both ways. It is easy to say "If I had only known, I would have done things differently," but it is never too late. Claiming your power and using your thinking in the most productive and creative ways now can help you make up for lost time. Become your own "thinking coach," and you'll be amazed at how quickly you'll see results.

> *I am what I think, and I have become what I have thought.*
>
> ~ Buddha (563–483 BCE),
> spiritual teacher from India

Remember Buddha's words. Look around you. Everything you see began when someone thought of it. The things around you came to you as a result of your thinking. Perhaps you have a car. At some point, you said to yourself, "I want one of those." Maybe you are married because you thought, "I like companionship, and I want more of it." You used your power of thought to own the ideas, because you first believed that you could have something or that something would make you happy. What you have in your life is there because you summoned it through your power of thought. This rule applies to the good stuff as well as the not-so-good stuff.

There is more good news: You can rethink and thus reclaim what you want in your life. Once you have used your power of thought, and you've clearly identified what you want, it will be summoned into your life. It will nudge away what it has come to replace.

> *Change your thoughts and change your world.*
> ~ Norman Vincent Peale (1898–1993),
> minister and author

Why do you need to know this important principle about thinking? The answer is because your life, your future, and the results you desire depend on knowing it and believing it. You can claim the power over your life.

I coauthored the book *Out of Your Mind* with my wife, psychologist Virginia Foster. With her permission, here are a few ideas from our book.

What if a genie appeared to you? Imagine he says that you could be happy and fulfilled in these three major areas of your life: prosperity, relationships, and health. He goes on to tell you that you can immediately start enjoying results and a feeling of being empowered. You might ask the genie: "What must I do? Where must I go? How much will this cost? How many years will it take?" You're fairly sure that the only way you could be fulfilled is by magic or immense luck.

Filled with curiosity, you ask, "How can I get the results I want in my life?"

The genie replies, "The formula is simple, but it is your responsibility to implement it."

Now you're totally mystified, so he continues. "Healthy, prosperous lifestyles, full of love and support, do not come about through fate and luck," he says. "Rather, they are a result of disciplined thinking." With those words of wisdom, the genie disappears.

You now have the answer in a nutshell: You can get what you want in life. You are the genie! The magic is to take charge of your thinking, take responsibility for your goals, and create the results. Your thoughts can either lift your spirits and encourage you onward, or they can bring you down and stop you in your tracks.

Imagine having the power to write an outline of how you think your day should be, but also having the power to hit the "escape" key so that you can start over and experience something better. This outline would resemble a shopping list. When I go to the grocery store I have a list. My list is on my computer. I have printed copies of it that contain the items I buy most often. My list is also a map of the store. When I go shopping I move quickly and always return home with every item I need.

Your outline of things "to do" and how you want your day to go can be like a map to help you move efficiently while making strides toward your goals. It would serve you best if the items on your list would be: to include a reminder to stay on top of your thinking by always looking for ways that it can be improved, to keep your goals in mind and be responsible for their accomplishment, and to look for ways your efforts are creating the results you desire. During the day, should a thought that is off-track spring up, know that you have the power to hit the "escape" key and correct your thinking, forgive yourself for letting it spring up, and praise yourself for noticing the potential delay it could have cause if gone unchecked. Then, check in with your list and stay on course.

Over the last decade, psychological research has pointed to the value of cognitive behavior therapy. (The word *cognitive* means "thought.") Such therapy is used to treat people with emotional disorders such as depression, anxiety, and phobias. Clients learn how to deal with unwanted feelings and troublesome emotions. When they have those feelings, they change the thoughts that cause the feelings.

In the same way, it is important to understand how your thinking creates results in your life. It's up to you to decide how to feel about events that happen. You can decide whether to have negative emotions or positive feelings. Remember that it's not how things are but what one thinks about how things are that creates either positive or negative feelings and behavior. It's not the actual event (or what someone else does or says) that causes joy or pain; it's the meaning we attach to the event. These emotions are based on what we think about life. These thoughts lead to feelings, and feelings can lead either to adaptive or maladaptive behavior.

For example, an acquaintance of ours became enraged when another driver cut him off on the freeway. He became so enraged that he forced the other car off the road and started a fight with the other driver. Why did he have such a dangerous reaction? The reaction came from his ideas about the situation. He thought that being cut off in traffic was catastrophic, and he thought that, in a situation like that, one must retaliate. These thoughts about the situation led to feelings of rage, and those feelings led to inappropriate and dangerous behavior.

> *One of the most important, but one of the most difficult things for a powerful mind is to be its own master.*
>
> ~ Joseph Addison (1672–1719),
> essayist, poet, and playwright

Our thinking creates our feelings, which are reflected in our behavior. Our behavior determines our overall life experiences. For example, imagine a woman named Joan who has this belief system: "No one likes me; I'm really unlovable." Unfortunately, Joan has to start working with Tom, who is temperamental and difficult with everyone. Joan personalizes this situation, believing that she is being persecuted by Tom. Joan gets angry and starts acting sarcastic and rude. Over a period of time, Joan's life becomes one of loneliness and rejection. This example shows how our thinking creates experience.

In cognitive behavior therapy, people are taught how to quickly change their thinking if they have uncomfortable feelings such as anger or frustration. How might Joan have changed things for the better? Choosing to see herself as a victim led to unhappiness. Instead, she could have realized that Tom was probably caught up in his own problems. When we have compassion for others, we can forgive them. That way, we do not have to waste any time judging others.

Cognitive behavior therapy is tremendously effective as a treatment for emotional problems, as it helps people learn to identify their thoughts and work on adjusting their thinking so they can reach the conclusions that are best for them, rather than fall into a way of thinking that creates the conflicts they are trying to overcome. As an ordained New Thought Unity minister, I've been using these same principles for years. Our thoughts act as magnets, attracting corresponding experiences. To be healthy, happy, and successful, we need to cultivate the maximum possible consciousness for being loving and compassionate. This kind of thinking will promote positive feelings, caring behavior, and an overall life experience that is healthy and fulfilling. The quality of our consciousness will determine how we interpret what we see and what reactions we have to what's going on around us.

Positive self-talk is quite helpful. This method can also be called affirmative self-talk. With this technique, you put into words the results you desire. You can write down the words, carry them with you, and repeat them often. Repeating these affirmations can keep you on track, and they can become the foundation for your thinking and thus produce the desired results.

If you're like me, you've used the power of affirmations in both positive and negative directions. Negative ones we've probably used are: "I know something is going to go wrong." "This is too good to be true." "I can't have what I want." Positive affirmations you and I have used most likely are: "I feel great, like I'm on top of the world." "I know I can do this." "I signed up for this, and I'm going to finish it."

I suggest you create your own affirmation for successful thinking. An example could be: "I am positive, loving, and compassionate. My thoughts determine my feelings, which lead to adaptive behavior, which determines my experience."

A diagram of how this Law of Mind Action works would look like this:

Think...Feel...Do...Have

A Thinking Evaluation

Understanding that what we think about we bring about is like saying, "What I'm conscious of shows up in my life." This is known as consciousness. Let's say that two people go on a picnic, for example. One is conscious of the ants, while the other is conscious of the beauty of the great outdoors. Which one is troubled because of the annoying ants, and which one doesn't even know the ants exist because he is conscious of the beauty and fresh air all around? What if the ant-conscious picnicker could ant-proof the picnic food and become aware of the bigger picture? Would he not become more pleasant to be around? Wouldn't he have good feelings about having recognized what he was thinking? Here's his formula:

THINK	He redirected his thoughts.
FEEL	He changed what he was feeling.
DO	He took the right action and ant-proofed the picnic food.
HAVE	He created the result of an enjoyable picnic.

Wouldn't he be more fun to be with now?

As we elevate the quality of our consciousness (which determines how we see and what reactions we have to what is going on around us) we elevate the results in our lives.

Perhaps as a way to see where you stand now, it might be helpful to ask yourself: "What am I thinking?" You could choose from any of these positive thoughts about your life:

Life is good.
Other people like me.
I enjoy prosperity.
I radiate health.

Or you can choose from any of these negative thoughts about your life:

Life is miserable.
I am not lovable.
There isn't enough money to go around.
I am illness-prone.

Feelings produced by and associated with the above positive thoughts might be joy, peace, contentment, love, and happiness. Feelings that are produced by and associated with the above negative thoughts probably are despair, hurt, depression, and disappointment.

Hopefully this evaluation will help you see that feelings always result from thinking either positive thoughts or negative thoughts. You must remember that to have positive feelings and results, you must think in ways that will create positive feelings, which will help you to direct your efforts toward your highest good. Your results come from your thoughts. Having the information from the first part of this evaluation (knowing that what we think about, we bring about in our life), it will be helpful to ask yourself: "What would my most positive thoughts be, and what would they sound like about what I want in my life?" In essence, "What would be the best way to think about what I want? And how would this thought present itself as my new affirmation?"

Asking yourself these questions will help you see what you need to be thinking and help you create a new replacement affirmation. As soon as you replace the old thought that no longer serves you with your latest creation, you'll notice a change in how you feel, and you'll be in touch with what you create.

Having this information and knowing that thoughts create feelings, it might be beneficial for you to visit your history and ask: "What positive feelings have I created in the past with my most positive thoughts?" You might recall a particular time at work when someone said something that was hurtful to you in the company of several coworkers. You remember your first reaction was to retaliate with a like kind of response. But, your thinking stepped in and helped you realize that such a reaction would not be in your best interest, especially because you did not want the others to see you behave in a way that was unflattering. In this example let's say your thinking helped you avoid experiencing and expressing the feelings that would damage your reputation with others. And your thinking helped you choose to create positive thoughts that created good results and feelings. Your self-talk then would sound something like: "Although they said hurtful things and I could have had a hurtful response, I choose to let their comments slide, which highlighted my reputation of being a better person in the presence of my coworkers." This example helps us see how beneficial it is to turn to your future and present thinking, and ask: "If my most positive thoughts and feelings are to materialize, how will this benefit me, and what will my behavior in the future look like?" And: "What experiences will I create as a result?"

Discipline of Thinking

Negative thinking brings about chaos and difficulty. A positive, loving approach cannot only help us realize our dreams, but it can also help us heal our bodies.

Training and learning to discipline yourself to be mindful of what you are thinking and how it will affect how you feel is a process that takes a little bit of time. So treat yourself with care and respect. When you realize you have fallen short of the mark, don't say, "You idiot! You were having negative thoughts again!" Instead, let your self-talk sound more like "Oops, you strayed off the path. Let's correct our position and call to mind the kinds of thoughts that serve you and keep you on track." Aligning yourself and making continual corrections is a sure way of training your thinking and creating a more disciplined mind.

Voodoo stories remind us of how powerful an idea can be. Followers of voodoo believe that the world is filled with demons and that they must continually take precautions to protect themselves from magical hazards. They believe that an enemy can attack them by sticking pins into a doll made in the victim's likeness. This belief can literally cause death. With this in mind, loving thoughts become even more attractive, and we can learn to develop a discipline of thinking where we simply refuse to indulge in negative thoughts.

Powerful thoughts create energy and magnetically draw corresponding experiences. I'm reminded of a friend of mine who was always expecting to be attacked while at home or out in public, jogging, or walking his dog. To protect himself, he mastered karate. During the time of our acquaintance, this friend was repeatedly attacked by burglars and muggers. He expertly defended himself with his martial arts. Once he became a hero when a restaurant where he was dining was held up. Singlehandedly, he apprehended two robbers with karate blows.

This example helps us understand that our enemies are never other people but simply what we're thinking. If we expect to be victimized or persecuted, we will create a condition where we are likely to attract exactly what we fear.

Let's look at another example. If we expect loneliness, rejection, and abandonment, each time someone is abrupt or distant, we'll indulge in thoughts like "Here it goes again. I'm a victim." Then, because our feelings follow our thoughts, we feel hurt and humiliated. We then behave in ways that push the other person away. Again, over time, the experience of life results in feelings of loneliness, rejection, and abandonment—exactly what we expected. Our thought is manifested as experience.

The sad part is that many parents raise children who expect loneliness, rejection, and abandonment based on how they were treated during childhood. Adults who were raised in dysfunctional families have to work especially hard at their discipline of thinking, in order to avoid perpetuating their childhood experience. Negative thinking causes a downward spiral.

Purity of Consciousness

Consciousness is simply the composition of our thoughts. Let's look at ways we can enhance our lives and achieve peace of mind through developing purity of consciousness. This requires discipline, yet it is an effort that can pay off richly. Using our uncharted territory analogy, the map to this location in our thinking looks like this:

Thought → Feeling → Behavior

What kinds of thoughts do you have when an unexpected bill comes? Have you ever thought, "I don't have enough money for extra expenses" or "I'm on a fixed income; I can't afford this"? What happens with this kind of thinking? You sabotage prosperity and create lack.

Let's look at an example: Many years ago, my wife's teenage son twisted his knee while surfing. He was in pain, so she took him to an orthopedist who promptly told her that her son needed an MRI. An MRI cost well over one thousand dollars at that time. Virginia suspected that the procedure was unnecessary, but she decided to follow the physician's advice. Her initial thoughts were: "I doubt very much there's anything wrong with his knee. This is going to be expensive, and it won't be covered by my health insurance."

She then caught herself thinking negatively and realized that these ideas would sabotage the flow of money into her life. She took hold of her thinking as she realized that the money would support the equipment and doctors and would make a contribution whether or not her son actually was injured. She began to affirm one of her favorite truths: "Money is constantly circulating into my life." She then went to the appointment, wrote her check for the MRI, and began to visit with others in the waiting room while she waited for the procedure to be done. In the process, her cheerful demeanor attracted visits from several doctors who subsequently referred patients to her psychological practice. The resulting income to her psychological practice was far greater than the expense of the MRI.

This is another example of how a thought ("Money is constantly circulating into my life") created an inner sense of peace and confidence. This confidence attracted others and motivated friendly behavior. The resulting experience was exactly what Virginia affirmed: "Money is constantly circulating into my life." (Happily, her prediction about her son was correct as well: Nothing was wrong with his knee.)

Over and over, we see that what we're thinking becomes reality in our lives. Through the process of thought we develop feelings. Feelings lead us toward behavior. Over time how we think, feel, and behave determines our life experience. Thus, we create what we've been thinking.

Positive ideas about love, prosperity, and health all result in feelings of happiness and abundance. When we're full of loving, positive feelings, we behave in ways that attract good things. Constantly thinking valid and rational thoughts manifests the results we desire.

A Case History in Thinking: Dorothy's Story

I first met Dorothy in the late 1980s, when she was in her 60s. My first impression of her was mixed. She was attractive, and, although she acted friendly, she had an unpleasant edge that pushed people away from her. Dorothy had a loving husband and a grown son, as well as a comfortable home filled with all the things a woman could want, and yet she conveyed emptiness and a sense of sadness with a twinge of anger. In situations where she was meeting new people, she tried hard to be warm and interested, but this sense of heavy sadness came through, and people avoided her. Her son had a life of his own, and he was busy. Her husband, who loved her dearly, did the best he could to show he cared for her, but he always felt frustrated because his caring never seemed to get through to her.

Dorothy found herself in a new place in her life when her husband died suddenly. His death was a big loss to her, and she grieved deeply. After a couple months of adjusting to his loss and learning to live on her own, she decided to take a sentimental journey and go back to her hometown and her roots.

She left California and flew to Ohio, rented a car, and drove to the little town where she was born and where her mother and sister were buried in the family plot in the town cemetery. After she checked into the Holiday Inn, she started to explore her old stomping grounds. She drove past her grandmother's house, around the town square (the kind with the courthouse in the middle), and past the movie theater where she got her first kiss. Then, after stopping at a flower shop, she went to the cemetery, where she placed flowers on the graves of her mother and sister.

With a little pair of scissors she took from her purse, Dorothy trimmed the overgrown grass around the edges of their headstones. As she brushed away the grass clippings, she noticed a mistake on her sister's headstone. The year of birth was incorrect. Instead of 1920, it showed 1918. Dorothy's sister had passed away a couple of years earlier, and Dorothy had made all the arrangements for her funeral and headstone. The headstone was ordered and installed after Dorothy returned to California, and she hadn't seen it. She had every reason to be upset as she went into the cemetery office to complain about this error.

The clerk said, "We are very careful about these kinds of things, but let me look at our records." She returned from a large filing cabinet with paperwork from the monument company and from the county clerk.

While she looked through the paperwork, Dorothy found the family agreement for the plot, and her mother and sister's death certificates. The clerk carefully read her sister's death certificate and said, "It states very clearly here that your sister was born in 1918."

"Well, there must be some mistake," Dorothy said, "because my sister and I are twins, and we were born in 1920."

The clerk replied, "This is an official document from the county clerk's office. I'm sure there is no mistake. Why don't I make you a copy of this, and you can take it to the county clerk's office and discuss the matter with them? I'll also make you a copy of your mother's birth certificate so you'll have it for your records."

Dorothy thanked her and left the cemetery office feeling confused and frustrated. She returned to her room at the Holiday Inn and pondered the paperwork. As she sat there, she didn't know that her life was about to change dramatically. After a restless night, she went to the county clerk's office. They assured her that there was no mistake. The year of her sister's birth was 1918, and the year of Dorothy's birth was 1920. Stunned, Dorothy went back to her motel room and sat in the big, comfortable chair. Then, she flashed back to a moment that she hadn't thought about in almost 60 years. She could vividly remember having ridden in an automobile between her mother, who was driving, and her sister, who sat by the window. All their earthly belongings were crammed into the backseat and the trunk. She distinctly remembered having heard her mother say, "We are on our way to a new life. Yes, we are moving to a new town, we'll live in a new place, and you'll start attending a new school. Best of all, you two will be twins! And I'll sew you new clothes, and you'll dress alike! We'll have so much fun! And when school starts, you'll both be in first grade."

Her mother then said to Dorothy's older sister, "I know you've already been to first grade, but you enjoyed it so much you can do it again. And Dorothy, you'll really like first grade, and you won't have to go to kindergarten." Then she said, "And your birthday will be the same day in March."

Dorothy's mother was so happy as she delivered this news that Dorothy and her sister shared her happiness without questioning the impact it could have on their lives.

When they moved into their new place, their mother got a job and the girls began first grade at the local school. It didn't take long for Dorothy to acquire the label of "the dumb one" because she was two years behind all the other students. Her sister was known as "the smart one" because she had already done the work once, and she was a year ahead of the other students. These labels stayed with these two girls all during their school years. Fortunately for Dorothy, she was pretty, and her good looks were an asset. She discovered early on that she was going to have to work very hard to keep up with the other students, which was hard to do with the addition of the stigma of being "the dumb one."

But she persevered, graduated from high school with her sister, got her first job, married her husband, and moved to California.

In the struggle to keep up, Dorothy had lost touch with what had happened in the car on the way to the new town and had suppressed it in her memory. It wasn't until that day at the motel, while looking at those birth certificates, that she discovered the memory of that experience.

After a sleepless night, she went directly to the cemetery. As soon as its big iron gates opened, she went to her mother's grave to have a "talk" with her. This was cathartic for Dorothy, and as she began to empty out her feelings of hurt, they turned into frustration and then anger while she expressed herself louder and louder. You could say she had a breakthrough. It was at this point that the funeral director approached her and said, "You are disrupting the peace, and we're having a graveside service in about an hour, and you'll have to leave." With that, Dorothy drove back to the motel, packed up her things, and returned home to California.

During the flight home, she had the opportunity to begin to put all of these events together, and she did the best thing she could do for herself: She found the good in the situation. She practiced the law of forgiveness toward her mother and realized that her mother didn't know the damage she would cause by living out this selfish fantasy of having twin daughters with the same birthday, and going to a new town and starting over. Dorothy also did some forgiveness work toward her sister for being the smart one, but most of all she found and gave herself credit for having done so well in spite of having started so far behind.

Dorothy said often, "I wasn't the dumb one! I must have

been pretty smart to find ways to keep up with the kids who were two years ahead of me."

The best part of Dorothy's story began at this time in her life. She realized that she had lived in a fog that someone else had created about whom she was and how smart she was. She realized she could reinvent herself rather than settle for someone else's description of her. When she took her life back, the change was wonderful to see. She had a new awareness of what a survivor she was, and how smart and capable she really was. This new awareness came through, and when she made new friends or associated with friends that she and her husband had together, she was perceived as a new person. That frustrated, almost angry feeling she used to give off had been replaced by a sense of worth and identity.

Dorothy not only found herself, but she also found time to be active in her neighborhood and in her church, and to help others. The possibilities she opened herself up to were inspiring, enlightening, and at times humorous. Once she said, "Out of habit I was reading my horoscope in the newspaper, and I realized I was reading the horoscope for March, and my birthday is in September. And all these years I've been reading the wrong horoscope!"

Eventually she joined a singles' dance club, met a delightful man, and fell in love. Nowadays she is in Paradise—Paradise, California, that is. She and her new husband live in a retirement community, they dance, they enjoy each other, they travel, and they share their time as volunteers in their community.

Dorothy's story has a happy conclusion because she discovered she had some thinking that needed to be changed, and she found the best way to rethink about herself and her life.

Dorothy's story illuminates the following points: Dorothy was told by the authority figures in her life how things were meant to be. She accepted what she was told, and she lived with it. Unfortunately, what she was told wasn't the truth about her, and it affected her negatively. Finally, after years of suffering, she awakened to the truth about herself and reclaimed her life.

Dorothy's experience can help us to examine current beliefs to see whether they are valid and whether we want to use them as tools to create our future. We can discover the truth about our own potential and reclaim our lives.

Once when I was at a car rental counter, I told the attendant something about how someday I'll do this or that, and she said, "Oh, that's an island." I asked what she meant, and she said, "Oh, haven't you heard of Someday Isle?"

I hadn't, but I have since created a map to the "I'lls" (Isles) of discovery we'll encounter as we go to and return from terra incognita at the conclusion of each chapter. These are the "I'lls" of: I'll Create, I'll Attract, and I'll Choose. There are also these islands: I'll Develop Interest and Belief, I'll Set Goals, I'll Experience the Law of Magnetism, I'll Move Slowly, and I'll Celebrate. We will also leave behind what I like to call the Harbor of Thought. That is, we won't return to the place from which we departed, because we'll have undergone so many changes that that place can no longer exist. I'd like you to think of the power of thought as a launching place rather than a destination.

Remember: It is from your thoughts that you form your world.

Your Map for Thinking

Begin by believing that your thinking is your internal guidance system and that it will move you to new heights.

Seek illuminating thoughts. This kind of thinking will spark ideas, and you will be inspired to action.

Expect results. You'll develop the awareness of what to do and how to develop the ability to do it.

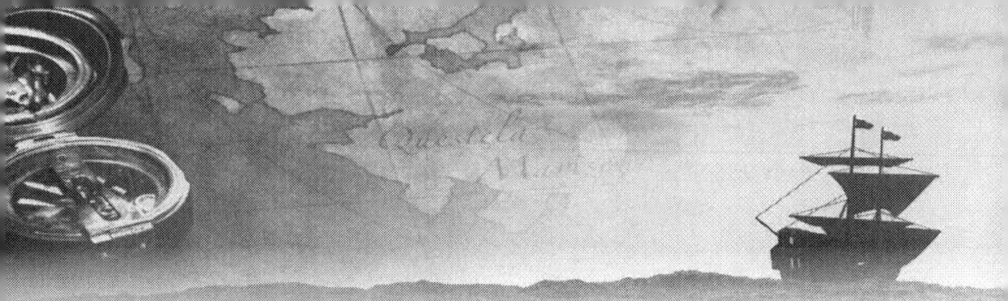

Chapter 3

You Can Create the Results You Desire

Even if you're on the right track, you'll get run over if you just sit there.

~ Will Rogers (1879–1935),
humorist and social commentator

ONE of the positive aspects of seeing what you want is that as you concentrate on what you're going to accomplish next in your life, your thoughts are lifted from the mundane and usual to the realm of possibility thinking. It's almost like being in love. As you're empowered with the ability to think about your goals, you abandon the kind of thinking that holds you back.

Researchers tell us we often learn best by hearing stories that illustrate a point. So, here's my story of how seeing what I wanted changed my life.

A dream come true for me was being accepted into the Unity School of Christianity Seminary in Lee's Summit, Missouri, just outside of Kansas City. On my way from California to Missouri, I was in an auto accident that delayed my arrival. When I arrived for registration, I was informed that all the accommodations for male students had been assigned and I'd be living in the girls' dorm.

This part wasn't a dream come true, because most of the "girls" were mature women who were old enough to be my mother. The three-story dorm had been a residence at one time, and each student had a private bedroom. There was a huge living room with a fireplace, a refrigerator next to a pay phone, and bathrooms down the hall. My room was spacious; I even had a desk for my typewriter, a closet, and a comfortable bed.

My school day began early with breakfast in the cafeteria, classes all morning, lunch, and then one more class until about 3 p.m. At this time, most of the students returned to their rooms to do homework. At the dorm, our routine followed a course that wasn't leading me to the results I wanted. I could easily finish my homework by 5 p.m., wander into the living room, and build a roaring fire in the big, stone fireplace. Within minutes, my housemates joined me. We'd order pizza and enjoy whatever refreshment we had donated to the refrigerator down the hall. As soon as the pizza was devoured we would visit and talk about the many spiritual ideas and principles presented to us in class that day.

We had good discussions and arguments, which was part of the learning process as we established our own belief systems. But after a while our discussions degenerated into conversations about our faculty and other students that wound up being critical and negative. I participated in these discussions as energetically as everyone else, and we all tried to outdo each other to be the funniest and most critical. Although displaying wit mixed with criticism seemed rewarding in the living room, the feelings I had upon returning to my room and going to bed weren't pleasant. I wasn't pleased with how I had behaved or by having used my time that way. And always, the following day when I saw faculty or fellow students I had spoken about so cleverly the night before, I felt uncomfortable.

After about two weeks of this routine, I returned to my room at the end of my school day and, as I was shutting the door, I said out loud, "I can't do this anymore. I'm not going to do my homework and then spend this evening in the living room putting people down, because that actually puts me down."

Then I asked myself, "Well, what are you going to do? You can't stay in your room. They'll think that you think you're better than they are or that you're unhappy with them."

I did not know that while I was looking for an immediate answer to the dilemma I was having, I was defining my life purpose. This is the moment when what I wanted started to appear. I can remember receiving impressions that supported my desire to do the right thing, which was to not sabotage my reputation or my education by sitting around talking about other people. My reply to my earlier question was this: "I don't know, but I know I can't stay here. I'll have to think of something, and I know some idea will come."

I knew I needed to make a plan.

Since then, each time I venture out into terra incognita and I reach this point where I ask the question "What do I want?" I often get many possibilities in reply. All I have to do is select the one that speaks to me the loudest. That day, some of the replies I received sounded something like this: "Well, you can go to the movies. You can go dancing. Or, you could get a job."

Of all these possibilities, getting a job rang the loudest bell. It had been years since I had applied for a job. My job as a minister's assistant had led to my desire to be a Unity minister, and the church I worked for had sponsored my entrance into the seminary. The job put me through college and gave me an income that met all my needs.

I asked myself, "If I got a job, what would I do?" Then, I had to put my creativity to work. As I searched for something that I could do after school and in the evenings, I had to inventory my skills. I realized that as a minister, I would be living a life of service. I thought about the jobs I had had. One of the first was as a carhop at an A&W Root Beer drive-in in Dallas when I was 13 years old. I had many pleasant memories of warm summer evenings, tips, burgers, and hot fudge sundaes. My thoughts then led me to decide that I would get a job as a waiter in a restaurant. The evening hours would fit my school schedule, and I could earn tips while learning about serving people and helping them have a good dining experience. This seemed to be the perfect answer, because it would keep me out of the "conversation pit," restore my reputation, and give me experience and income.

I was already dressed for an interview, in my campus attire of a crisp white dress shirt and tie with slacks. So I got into my car and started driving toward Kansas City. After so many years of having had the same job, applying for a job was scary, but I drove forward anyway. After thinking "Where will I start, and what will I do?" my burning desire to do the best thing I could for my school reputation helped me see myself serving people as a waiter. I was driving through my old world to break through into a new world.

I like to be surrounded by beautiful things. I thought, "I'd like to be a waiter in a very fancy restaurant." The fanciest restaurant I knew was atop the 52-floor Commerce Towers Building in downtown Kansas City. Although I did not know if a job was available, I decided I'd go there and tell them, "I'm Arthur Hammons, and I've come for the waiter's job."

As I drove on, I saw myself being hired that very afternoon. I saw myself learning the skills to be a waiter in an elegant restaurant. I saw myself making a good income, and, best of all, I saw myself pulling away from the habit of criticizing others and sabotaging my future. I held my imminent success in my mind, and I practiced my speech repeatedly: "I'm Arthur Hammons, and I've come for the waiter's job."

I had been to the Commerce Towers with a friend during

summer school while training to become a licensed Unity teacher. We had enjoyed a drink in the bar, so I was somewhat familiar with the restaurant and knew that it had various-themed rooms: the German Room, the Italian Terrace, the Cantina Bar, and the French Room. I would have been happy to work in any of them, but the French Room was the most elegant. So on the drive, I envisioned myself working in that room, serving people in the best of their circumstances who were beautifully dressed, well-mannered, and generous tippers.

I parked in the underground lot and took the elevator to the 52nd floor, practicing my acceptance speech each step of the way. Once I arrived at my destination, I drew a deep breath, squared my shoulders, stood up straight, and went through the 12-foot-high doors into the business office, where the receptionist looked up and said, "Can I help you?"

I replied, "I'm Arthur Hammons, and I've come for the waiter's job."

She depressed a button on the intercom box on her desk, leaned forward, and said, "Mr. Bath, Arthur Hammons is here for the waiter's job." Then she said to me, "Mr. Bath will be right out."

Mr. Bath came out of his office, and, without looking at me or slowing as he passed, he said, "Come with me." I followed him out of the office and down the hallway, through a stainless-steel maze of countertops and pots and pans, through doors that went into the public entrance—and into the French Room!

Mr. Bath approached the tuxedo-clad maître d and said, "This is Arthur Hammons. He's come for the waiter's job." Then he turned and left.

The maître d extended his hand and said, "I'm Louie. Let's go upstairs and get your tuxedo. Then I'll introduce you to the rest of the team, and we'll set the tables and be ready to open at five. I'd like you to observe our headwaiter, Hino, as he waits on a couple of tables, and then I'll give you your own tables. Our menu is small, and it's written in French, and most people can't read it, so you'll need to be able to speak enough French to read the menu to them by tomorrow evening."

That's what Louie was saying to me, but as we went upstairs to get my tuxedo I was saying to myself, over and over, "My God, I got the job. My dream has come true. This is really happening." I was glad that I was wearing my crisp white shirt as I slipped into tuxedo pants, a waiter's jacket, and a long white apron. I replaced my necktie with a bowtie, and I was ready to go except for one thing: The next day I started to learn conversational French in preparation for my new job.

But I didn't need to know French that night; I was only observing and helping. I joined Hino, Louie, and the busboy and busgirl in setting tables and getting ready for our evening guests. The French Room was really beautiful, with its tall ceiling and panoramic windows adorned with puffed-silk draperies. An oriental carpet that I learned had been woven especially for the room covered the floor, and in its center was a round kitchen island. This wasn't the type of kitchen island you see in home kitchens; this kitchen island was the room's focal point. It was where all the cooking and sautéing happened, and where all the sauces were made and the flambé dishes flamed. From the high ceiling hung four crystal chandeliers that at one time had been in the St. Louis Opera House.

My duties as a waiter were to welcome our guests, take their cocktail and wine orders, read the menu to them in French, and describe each entrée, appetizer, and dessert before taking their order. One of our specialties was our Caesar salad, which we tossed tableside in a large, silver bowl. This was usually followed by escargot, French onion soup, or quiche Lorraine. Our 7-foot-tall (with hat) chef would prepare the entrées with a lot of drama and flair. When our guests finished their meal, we'd present them with an elegant array of French pastries and confections from our dessert cart, followed by coffee. The people I served were almost always friendly and happy, celebrating either an anniversary or a romantic night on the town. It was always fun to go to work, and our guests were generous tippers.

Looking back on this experience, I'm glad that it started when I asked, "What do I want?" received the answer, and could vividly see the results I wanted. I can still feel my hand on the doorknob, and I remember the breakthrough I made for myself into the life I had gone to seminary to create.

The return on the investment I made within myself paid off in many ways for the rest of my school year. Not only did I stay out of trouble, but I also had a reputation of being a hard-working student who had a job and no time to be involved with unworthy activities. My experiences as a server put me in touch with my customers' needs, and I learned how to help them in times of celebration as well as when things went wrong or they were unhappy. I was able to transfer many of the lessons I was learning at my job into my class assignments.

The story gets even better. Another benefit of having a good reputation with my professors came about when the Silent Unity Prayer Ministry at our seminary needed a student minister to answer prayer requests on the 24-hour phone line. This was the oldest continual prayer service in the United States. It was started by the founders of the Unity movement and is one of the most revered activities of the Unity School of Christianity. To work there was truly an honor, given to only the best and most hardworking students at the seminary. I was selected to fill this two-nights-a-week position, which no student minister had been allowed to fill for seven years because a past student had responded unkindly to a caller. I had the best of both worlds. One world was filled with crystal chandeliers, fancy-dressed people, and elegant parties. The other offered the opportunity to help people who were often desperate and upset because of an emergency. I trust that this story will inspire you to realize that you have the power of thought and, by using it, you can create the results you desire. The combination of your thoughts and creativity will stimulate the Law of Attraction, which will offer a catalog of possibilities and inspiration. Then, as I did, you'll have the opportunity to see what you want and bring it into your life. After I had been working in the French Room for a couple of weeks, during our evening routine of setting the tables, Louie asked me, "Which restaurant did you work in in New York City?"

Confused, I replied, "I've never been to New York City."

"Didn't Sam from the Red Pony restaurant over on Twelfth Street send you here?" Louie asked.

"I don't know what you're talking about," I replied, outright befuddled.

And Louie said, "On the day you started work here, my friend Sam called me and asked me if I needed a waiter. I said yes, and he said he had a really experienced guy from New York City who was looking for a job, and he'd send him right over."

The memory of my coming into the office that day with my "I'm Arthur Hammons, and I've come for the waiter's job" speech returned. And the idea of taking the job of someone who really needed it troubled me deeply.

I asked Louie if he'd come with me to Mr. Bath's office, and he did. There, we asked Mr. Bath if any other guys had come in to apply for the waiter's job that day. Mr. Bath assured us that no one had come in looking for work in weeks. My vision of seeing what I wanted was so intense, I was so sincere about wanting the job, and my motives for having it were so clearly defined that the way was made clear for me. The way was paved with possibilities that I made the most of through seeing what I wanted. When you see what you want and believe that you can have it, it will be yours.

> *Creativity often consists of merely turning up what is already there.*
>
> ~ Bernice Fitz-Gibbon (1894–1982), advertising executive

The next step in charting your way to success, health, wealth, and all you've ever dreamed of is to realize that you are the creator of your results. Everything you've experienced and all the things you have were created by you. You drew them to you. All your future results will also be created by you. Unpredictable and often unfortunate things sometimes happen. Sometimes things just go wrong. It doesn't sound very caring to say "They created that" when the circumstances were random or they were at the wrong place at the wrong time. However, you can create what you want, and when things pop up randomly or you encounter delays, you can use your power to rethink and take all the responsibility you can. Claiming your creative responsibility in conjunction with the accomplishment you are seeking empowers you to work with the cards you've been dealt to create the best possible outcome.

Looking back, you might remember a time when you didn't have clear intentions, and you didn't know exactly what you wanted, and you experienced results that were less than desirable. Maybe you failed to ask for a promotion and saw a coworker get the job you wanted. Or perhaps the girl you were in love with married someone else because you never got up enough courage to propose to her. Or you didn't enter that talent show at school, and people who couldn't sing as well as you won the prizes. "Did I create that?" you ask. Ruling out those untimely interruptions mentioned above, you did create it. Somebody created it. If it wasn't you, then who? Somehow, on some level, you thought, "I need this," or "I'll get this," or "What if this happens?" In one way or another, you said, "This is my ticket to the results I want." Perhaps some part of your consciousness knew that if you had this experience it would add information to your collection, move you forward, and deepen your ability to reach your goals. Even if things go wrong or are interrupted, you can work around them and create the desired outcome. Perhaps the following story will be a helpful illustration of this concept.

My first marriage was to a woman with whom I thought I was truly in love. I wanted love in my life, I wanted companionship, and I wanted to have children. Together we had two sons, and after eight years of being married we dissolved our partnership.

Breaking up truly is hard to do. During this deeply challenging time, I kept asking myself, "Why did I create this?" After months of soul-searching I found my answer.

I wanted love in my life, and I created it. The experience was good for me because it taught me a lot about love, and it educated me on how to recognize lasting, committed love. It also trained me how to be better at giving and receiving love.

I also wanted companionship, and I created it. The experience was good for me because it helped me define what deep, lasting companionship really is.

I also wanted children, and we created two of them. The experience of being a father has been one of my life's best opportunities to demonstrate love, to grow and work on my own issues, to learn, and the list goes on.

I might not have chosen these specific developments, but my general needs had my creative forces behind them, and they became manifest. I believe they became real in my life because something deep within me knew what I needed as well as what I wanted.

The next page of my love life began when I had healed from the past and decided that I wanted love and companionship in my life again. This time I had some experience that helped me create the love I wanted. I did a better job the second time around. Along with an evolved awareness of love came a matching awareness of companionship, which I used to satisfy that want. Healing of the past followed on a higher level, because I could forgive myself for choices I had made that did not seem to serve me at the time but that led to my highest good. Hindsight helped me see that I did create the events of my life and that they brought the results I longed for and so much more. All I had been through was worth it, and I was better for the experience. This is where we apply the principle that teaches us to "throw out the experience, and keep the lesson."

Now that we're discussing concepts that can be roadblocks to our success, let's investigate this idea: People create their conditions; conditions don't create people.

It might have looked as though you were in the right place at the right time, but you created the place and time and drew them to you because of the power you have to create and the need for that power to be expressed. The same applies to the other side of the coin—being at the wrong place at the wrong time. Think of the many heroes who have stepped forward to rescue someone. Were they in the right place at the right time, or was it in their makeup to be a hero?

How many victims have been caught up in something bad? Was that the wrong place or the wrong time for them, or was it in their makeup to be a victim?

Why not stop and think about the alternatives and possibilities? What if every time was the right time, and every place was the right place, and you were there to experience the best you could while stepping forward to build the life you want?

A better way to think about any situation you find yourself facing is having an awareness that reflects this statement: "This situation isn't happening to me; I am happening to this situation. I bring my best to it, and it brings out the best in me. I simply will not have it any other way."

Whether you agree or disagree with the ideas you've created in your present situation, you shouldn't block yourself from claiming your creative power and using it wisely to manifest what you want in your future. You have already established your power by declaring that you can choose which thoughts will serve you. Now take the next step and combine that power with your power to create.

> *Imagination is more important than knowledge.*
> ~ Albert Einstein (1879–1955),
> author of the theory of general relativity

One day, just for fun, I was sitting in my living room looking at our coffee table. I asked myself, "How can I think differently about this coffee table?" My first thought was that there was nothing new I could discover about it. Then all of a sudden, it hit me. I realized that our coffee table is decaffeinated! I *could* think about it differently.

Feeling inspired, I went down the hall to our guest room and discovered that the twin beds are fraternal. Then I went to the knife drawer in the kitchen and found that our meat thermometer isn't oral!

This shows that you can think and create an awareness you never had before, and change your perspective on just about everything.

Here is a list of some important beliefs about your powers of thinking to claim for yourself. Read the list and incorporate these beliefs into how you want to live your life. They'll help you master your thinking and create the results you're dreaming of.

You are the creator of your world.

> You limit yourself when your mind is choked with perceived limitations, false beliefs, and a lack of interest.

Your thoughts will attract exactly what you need.

We systematically draw people, places, and circumstances into our lives.

Our thoughts eventually become our reality.

Thoughts become actions. Actions are three-dimensional thoughts.

Through our thoughts, we give life to our world.

You have the power to create or destroy.
Your mind is your most wondrous creation.
Your mind knows only the limits you use to hold it back.

Next is a list of several important beliefs to cultivate about how to direct your creativity and acquire what you want. Study this list and incorporate it into your "crew of abilities," so it's there to help you as you navigate through terra incognita.

Clearly see what you want to create.

Thoughts held in mind produce after their kind.
We move in the direction of our thoughts.
Where you are looking is where you are headed.
Where you put your vision is where you put your attention and where you end up.
You always create an exact outer replica of the inner idea.
This is called the Law of Mind Action.
You are a rendition of your persistent ideas.
You produce according to the thoughts you hold.
The thoughts you feed the most grow to be the strongest.

Believe in your powers of thought and creativity.

Learn to find your center.

> Tell yourself the real story about your thoughts and feelings.
> Identify yourself as a "feeler" or a "thinker," and remind yourself that thoughts come before feelings.
> Are you driven by your emotions or your thoughts?
> Attach an emotion to a thought, and the thought becomes motivated to take action and become alive.

When thoughts and feelings reach critical mass, they can be transformed to a level that prompts us to action.

Once you're aligned with the two lists about thought and creativity, you'll arrive at a place where you'll want to synchronize your thoughts and feelings to prepare to do the work of creating what you want. Then you'll want to ask yourself these important questions:

> Am I really interested in developing the consciousness to have what I want?
> Do I really believe I can have what I want?
> Am I willing to do the work of evaluating my thinking, stimulating my creativity, and drawing a clear vision of the steps to take in manifesting what I want?

Develop an Attitude of Complete Responsibility for Your Life

Psychological Monographs, a book written in 1966 by researcher Julian B. Rotter, taught us that people have two ways of looking at their successes or failures. Some people have what we call an external locus of control. They locate the control over what happens to them as being outside themselves. They attribute many of the reasons for the events in their lives to fate and luck.

By contrast, another group of people have an internal locus of control. They believe the reasons for their harmony in life, or lack of it, are due to their own abilities and efforts. They're responsible for the outcome of whatever they attempt. If a plan fails, they try to learn from what happened and develop new plans. They don't waste time or cause confusion by blaming circumstances or other people. If another person gets in the way, they take responsibility for choosing to be involved in that relationship. Their locus of control is within.

Logic dictates that the only way to manifest the lifestyle you want is to look at life with an internal locus of control—to take complete responsibility for the quality of your life and your future.

You might be thinking, "That's fine for you to say, but you don't know my boss," or "If you had children like mine, you wouldn't say that."

It's important to emphasize that all the major religions of the world have taught us not to judge. There's a good reason for this: Judgment gets in the way of taking responsibility. If we judge others and blame them for our difficulties, we block ourselves from creating the results we want.

When we aren't responsible, we align our results with defeat, frustration, and anxiety. These feelings are perpetuated by the idea that the external is in control. It is not true that what happens to you shapes your life. It is true that how you think about what happens to you shapes your life. Taking responsibility for your thinking is the starting point.

Taking responsibility is a mark of character and maturity that each of us can expand on. Each of us is a work in process—unfolding and expanding as we enlarge our area of experience and expertise. Claiming responsibility, ceasing all criticism, and knowing that no one will come to rescue us from the responsibility we have to ourselves is the starting point for being all we can be and experiencing fulfillment in our lives. When we fall into the common trap of blaming others, we get in the way of creating results. Don't worry about other people and circumstances; simply decide what you want. If you have a clear vision of success in your particular career, and if you develop that vision and believe in it, you can overcome the obstacles in the way.

By contrast, without this quality of responsibility, you might think, "I can't have the career I want because my boss doesn't support me." This idea will stop you before you ever get started on the vision. Begin with the vision clearly in mind, and the boss will become only an obstacle blocking your way to achieving your goal. You might decide to be assertive and see if you can get more cooperation, or you might change companies or even start your own business. It's when you develop your vision, taking complete responsibility for your life without blaming others, that you're on your way to manifesting the results you want.

A Case History in Creating What You Want: Annette's Story

Annette was quite attractive, with her hair pulled back in a neat little bun and a pretty face. She reminded me of Nefertiti, but her most outstanding quality was her strong yet graceful body. When I first met Annette she appeared to be in her 60s. We were at a cocktail party, and she was wearing a little black dress that showed off beautiful skin tightly wrapped around feminine muscles. In our getting-to-know-you conversation, I asked her, "What do you do?" I'll never forget her response. She placed an open hand over her heart and said, almost seductively, "I'm a dancer."

Over the course of many years I was privileged to hear Annette's story. From what I understand, Annette was born on her toes; her first steps were dance steps. As a child, she used to dance in the sunlight that streamed through the windows in her Louisiana home. Unfortunately, her loving parents never saw this beautiful child of theirs. They were blind, but they always knew how special she was, and, although they never saw her dance, they had unwavering love for her. She showed so much promise as a dancer that they put her in dance classes. She was always the star of the recitals and gained countywide fame dancing at church potlucks, fairs, and money-raising events. Annette's talent was so obvious that her dance instructor encouraged her parents to send Annette to dance school in New York City. This was a far-fetched dream, because the money for such an education was nonexistent, especially for a sightless couple who made brooms for a living.

Annette was resourceful and determined, and these qualities had always brought her the results she desired. Having a passion for being in dance school and for living in New York City, she told her parents she was going to write for a scholarship and that she had a letter of recommendation from her dance instructor. While she and her family waited for a response from the dance school, she talked constantly about going to the big city. She knew that her chances of being accepted at the school were slim, because all she had were the application and the recommendation letter. The requirements for admission said that she needed to be there in person and audition to even be accepted as a student. She knew that her parents couldn't afford it and that they would never allow their 16-year-old girl to go to New York City. So Annette took a blank piece of paper, unfolded it in front of her parents, and said, "I've been accepted, and I'm supposed to leave immediately for New York City."

Her parents explained that they only had enough money for a one-way ticket, but Annette assured them the school had promised a place to live with several other girls and that jobs were plentiful. A bus ticket was purchased, and the next thing she knew, she stood in front of the acceptance committee at the school.

Her audition performance was flawless. The faculty was impressed. She was accepted.

At the bulletin board in the hallway outside the audition room, she met her future roommates, and they pooled their resources so the six of them could live in a studio apartment nearby. One of the girls had a job at a delicatessen, and she said Annette could work with her there. Another of the girls was the envy and inspiration of the other roommates, because she had a job with the New York City Ballet. While the other girls headed off to their jobs, she went to the rehearsal halls at the Metropolitan Opera.

Annette's daily routine was to dance several hours, work hard at the deli until late at night, get some sleep, and wake up in time to get back to the dance school the next day. She was happy and was constantly creating the future she wanted. While working long hours to support herself, she attended grueling dance classes each day. One day while Annette was working at the deli the door burst open, and in came the roommate who danced at the Metropolitan. "Annette, you've got to come with me right now," she said. "One of the girls in the chorus has an injury, and we need a replacement for tonight's performance. Come quickly."

Annette looked at her boss with big, pleading eyes, and he gestured toward the door. She yanked off her apron and took off for the theater with her roommate.

"Does this mean I'm going to be on the stage of the Metropolitan Opera?" Annette asked, still in shock.

"Yes," her friend replied.

"But I don't know what dance we're doing or any of the steps—"

"You'll be fine," the friend said. "Tonight's performance is the opera *Samson and Delilah,* and we're Delilah's handmaidens. There *are* no steps to this dance; it's all improvisational. All you need to do is swirl around, do a few pirouettes, and sprinkle flower petals in Delilah's path. Just do what the other girls do, and you'll be fine."

Annette's dream was coming true! She had always envisioned herself doing what she loved to do the most—to dance—on the stage of the Metropolitan Opera. Of all the stages to be dancing on, this was the most prestigious. Her excitement grew while she stepped into her costume and applied her makeup with all the other dancers. As she told them how nervous as she was, they assured her that what she had to do was easy. "We just dance out with Delilah and act like her handmaidens. We're in the first act, and that's when she meets her boyfriend, Samson. We're not in the second act. But in the third act, we accompany her as she visits him in the prison scene. Just think of yourself as her handmaiden, do what the rest of us do, and you'll be fine."

Everything did go fine for the first act. Annette felt the heat of the lights and the presence of the audience while she swirled and danced to the music of the orchestra welling from the pit below. She was in dancer's heaven. The first act ended without a hitch. She took a break during the second act and prepared for the third act and finale.

The third act began, and she stepped out on the stage dressed in a beautiful costume, as were Delilah and the rest of the dancers. But the stage, which had been so colorful and cheery in the first act, was now dreary and dark. When she saw Samson, he had also drastically changed since the first act. Now, he looked as though he'd been hit by a truck. Annette thought, "Did he get a haircut during the second act?"

Then, just as in the first act, Samson sang to Delilah, and she sang to him. Annette had never been to Sunday school, and she didn't know the story of Samson and Delilah. She was simply caught up in the moment, the pageantry, the music, and the fact that her dream of being on the stage at the Metropolitan Opera was coming true.

Among what seemed a hundred cast members on the stage, Annette watched while Samson embraced Delilah, and they sang their romantic duet. Then he stepped away from her, and, with his chains dragging on the floor, he stepped up some scenery steps and stood between two pillars. Then he sang his triumphant ending and pushed the pillars apart. This caused all the scenery to collapse, and huge pieces of what appeared to be stone and heavy timbers started falling from above.

Everyone on the stage screamed in terror and began to run off stage. Pandemonium erupted. Annette found herself frozen, center stage, and as the others fled, she didn't know which way to turn. It seemed that either direction was too far to safety, and she thought her life was about to end.

Then, just as the curtain was about to close, Annette saw an opening that she thought might allow her to exit in time to avoid being hit. With a scream, she leaped through the opening—and plunged into the orchestra pit. The curtain closed, and the final notes of the orchestra ended with a crescendo.

Annette stood, and was surprised to find she was not hurt. Then, to her astonishment, the grand curtains opened, and there were Samson, Delilah, the corps de ballet, the chorus, and the extras taking their bows. Not one of them was hurt. Realizing at last that the big end-of-the-world scene was simply a part of the show, she was mortified.

That night, as she and her roommate and the other girls of the chorus were leaving the theater, the mistress of the ballet said to Annette, "Young lady, be in my office at 8 a.m. tomorrow."

Annette knew this meant her days at the Metropolitan would be over before they had had a chance to begin. After a sleepless night, promptly at 8 a.m., she appeared before the mistress of the ballet. The ballet mistress said, "I don't know what you were thinking last night as you leaped into the orchestra pit. I was ready to let you go on the spot." Then she asked, "Have you seen today's headlines?"

"No, I haven't," Annette replied.

Then the mistress held up a copy of the *New York Times*. The headlines said, "Opera Performance" and "Best Ever." The mistress explained to Annette that the article had mentioned a certain ballerina who had made the ending scene "very convincing" by leaping into the orchestra pit. She then went on to say that this kind of publicity from the newspaper and Annette's drama would mean sold-out performances for the rest of the opera's run.

Then the ballet mistress said, "I have good news, and I have bad news. The good news is I'm going to keep you in the corps de ballet. The bad news is you have to leap into the orchestra pit Friday night, Saturday night, and at the Sunday matinee."

Annette's dream had come true, and the spotlight she saw herself in was real. This shows the power of creativity and of always keeping your dream in mind.

Annette stayed with the Metropolitan Ballet and appeared in many performances. She exhibited so much talent that she became a principal with the company and went on to perform on stages worldwide. She met royalty, musicians, writers, directors, designers, playboys, tycoons, and stage-door johnnies. She received bundles of long-stemmed roses, jewelry, party invitations, and numerous marriage proposals. She went from living in a tiny studio to a lovely residence in New York City. She was also generous toward her parents, taking care of them in their old age and seeing to it that they were comfortable. Although they never saw their daughter perform, they attended many of her performances.

At the peak of her career, Annette realized that it was time for her to retire and give younger talent the opportunity to experience all the wonderful things she had experienced. She retired and became a member of the Metropolitan's teaching faculty. There, she had the opportunity to pass her skills on to others, which was her way of giving back.

In the next chapter of her life she opened a dance studio and taught dancing to youngsters. This, too, was enormously fulfilling. Eventually, as she tired from the many tasks that come with running a business, Annette passed the business on to someone else and devoted her time to being a volunteer teacher to children who were less fortunate and couldn't afford ballet school. Again, she was giving back to show her appreciation for all the good she had experienced in her life.

One evening, while going home from a dance recital in Harlem, she was run over by a hit-and-run driver. Her injuries were extensive. When she got to the hospital, the doctors did everything they could to save her life. Their efforts were successful, although Annette remained unconscious for several days. When she regained consciousness, the doctors explained to her that while she was being taken to the hospital, her identification and handbag had been lost, and the hospital staff had no idea of her name, age, or occupation. She replied, "I'm a dancer, my name is Annette, and I am 82 years old."

With gasps, the nurses replied, "You must still be under the influence of drugs, because you couldn't possibly be 82 years old. We've been taking care of you for the past several days, and we know your body, and you don't have the body of an 82-year-old woman. You have the body of a woman in her 50s. And because you're in such great shape, your body saved your life. Anyone else being hit by a car and lying there in the dark for as long as you did couldn't have survived such an accident."

And Annette repeated, "I'm a dancer."

Annette had created the career she dreamed of when she started dancing in those sunbeams, she lived a life of performance that inspired and entertained thousands of people, and she gave back to her community from the overflow her career had created in her life. While she was doing all this, she was building a body that served her all her life. Not only did this strong body serve her, but it saved her life.

After mending from her accident, she went back to work volunteering and teaching with passion. Her story is a testament to creativity. She knew exactly what she wanted, and she moved toward the result she desired without letting the "in between" frighten or discourage her.

Annette is one of my heroes because her story weaves together the principles of creating what you want.

Your Map to "I'll Use Creativity to Reach My Destination"

Now that you know you can have results, let's look at the formula for doing so. It consists of these steps:

Develop an attitude of complete responsibility for your life.
Identify yourself as the one responsible for creating what you want.
Decide that you have the interest and belief that you can have what you want.
Be prepared to do the work required.
Anticipate the inspiration and delivery of your catalog of possibilities and beliefs.
Be prepared to put your goals in writing.
Develop the capacity to visualize the result and create a schedule for what you need to do.

These steps will be discussed in future chapters.

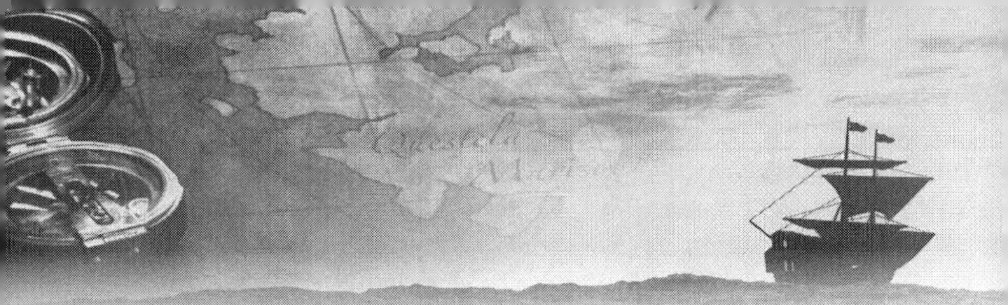

Chapter 4

Attract Your Catalog of Possibilities: Decide What You Want

Hold a picture of yourself long and steady enough in your mind's eye, and you will draw toward it.

~ Napoleon Hill (1883–1970),
motivational speaker and author

IN this chapter, I'll introduce you to the wonder and magic of the Law of Attraction. I like to think of this next step in the process of charting your way to all you desire as the one where you receive your catalog of possibilities. Once you're convinced that your thoughts and thinking are powerful, and you've directed them to claiming your power to create what you desire, you've reached the point where you attract your own catalog of impressions of what you can create and have.

This catalog is uniquely yours. It's not like the Neiman Marcus catalog; it's better! And the models who are pictured aren't other people; they're you. The items are there for you to see and choose. Some goals are very reasonably priced, while others appear extremely expensive with regard to the time and work they will take to accomplish. I particularly like this step because the visions my catalogs have revealed to me have been so clear and inviting that I couldn't resist their invitation to work hard and have them appear as reality in my life. Summon your catalog with thought and creativity, and, as it arrives, be prepared to be inspired and amazed. A few years ago a best-selling book titled *The Secret* swept the nation with information about the Law of Attraction. It was everywhere. Oprah shared it on her television show, and copies flew off the shelves in bookstores. Although it is not the originator of the concept, the book is a helpful tool for understanding this law.

As you master the Law of Attraction, there are some things to remember. One is to enjoy the feeling of rising to a new level of awareness. You'll feel a flow of energy and creativity that invites you to leave your routine thinking and accept the invitation to think more creatively. I think you'll also feel a familiar tug that says, "Don't go there; that's too much work; don't make waves; leave well enough alone." I expect the invitation to increase and to make your move to the next step in your life will be more intriguing. Yes, there will be emotional and physical costs, but the rewards will be worth the effort.

> *People who ask confidently get more than those who are hesitant and uncertain. When you've figured out what you want to ask for, do it with certainty, boldness and confidence.*
>
> ~ Jack Canfield (b. 1944),
> motivational speaker and author

When your catalog arrives, look through it and enjoy the presentation of all the many possibilities you've attracted. Immediately, you'll see how powerful your thinking and creativity are. Feeling this power, you'll then direct it to manifest your desires—desires not only for your material gain, but for accomplishments that reflect your ability to create.

Maybe you can write a poem, or a short story, or even a novel. What if your book were published? What if it became a best-seller? Not only do such accomplishments pave the way to your future, they're so predominant in the present that they block out your past by presenting and supporting not the new you, but the *now* you. Once you achieve these results, you can't go back to living on a lesser level. You'll be like a balloon that, once inflated, can't go back to its former shape.

Once you accept delivery of your catalog of possibilities and beliefs, your subscription is set, and you'll be receiving such catalogs for the rest of your life. They keep adjusting with your needs. You ensure this process by nourishing your thoughts with the anticipation that ideas and inspiration are yours to develop.

A Case History in Attracting Your Possibilities, Deciding What You Want, and Doing The Work: Ed's Story

Ed was born in Long Beach, California, to a couple who failed at parenting. His parents were never home, they didn't have consistent jobs, and the members of the household were on their own to eat, care for themselves, and get where they needed to be. Ed was a good-looking kid with bright blue eyes and a shock of blond hair. He was sharp and eager to learn, but school was a struggle. It was a struggle to get there, find something to make for lunch or do without, and then come home to an empty and often-unlit and cold house. This was at a time when child protective services were less developed than they are now, and teachers weren't as involved and aware as they are today.

With no supervision at home and time on his hands, Ed was

drawn in by older kids who influenced his desire to act grown-up and enticed him to do petty acts of crime. Before long Ed was in trouble. The trouble reached school and followed him everywhere. By the time he was 16, the police in Long Beach knew Ed well. Once a police officer told him he probably wouldn't reach the age of 18 if he pursued the path he was on, and the officer suggested that Ed get out of town and find a better life. At this point Ed received his first catalog of possibilities and beliefs. He knew that he needed to change or suffer extremely negative results.

After dropping out of school, he took all the possessions he had—a couple of shirts, a jacket, a pair of jeans (all black), his only pair of running shoes, some underwear and socks, and a Bible someone had given him—and left for someplace, anyplace better. He would have said goodbye to his parents, but as usual it had been days since he had seen them. At the nearest freeway, he stuck out his thumb. Someone picked him up, drove him north, and dropped him off at a gas station. This began a pattern in which Ed used his winning smile and good looks to get a job sweeping or cleaning windows and restrooms in exchange for a Coke and a candy bar. Then it was back to the road, thumb in the air, until the next drop-off, usually at another gas station.

Eventually Ed reached Oregon, where he charmed his way into a job cleaning around a roadside cafe and doing yard work in exchange for a hamburger and a place to sleep. The owner, an older woman, took a liking to Ed and perceived him as an honest and hardworking kid who had had a rough start in life. As their friendship grew, she let him move into a small back room at the cafe and out of the drafty shed by the Dumpster. She was right about Ed. He was a diligent worker, and before long he had cleaned every surface and window, made many much-needed repairs, and covered most of the place with fresh paint. The woman's kindness brought her a newly refurbished establishment, which attracted new customers to enjoy her tasty food, and a new friend. This resulted in her hiring Ed to help her in the kitchen.

The Law of Attraction was working its magic, because Ed was thinking and acting. He wasn't in trouble, and he felt good about his life. His desire for more good in his life attracted more items in his personal catalog of possibilities and beliefs.

Usually on Friday evenings, an elderly couple frequented the cafe for its fish-and-chips special. By then Ed was washing dishes and bussing tables. The couple, who were friends with the owner, eventually became acquainted with Ed. They often stayed after the other customers left, and they would join the owner and Ed in dessert and long conversations. Seeing what a bright, capable, and caring young man Ed was, and knowing that he'd gained the trust of the cafe owner, the couple invited him to come to their ranch for dinner. This invitation became a routine every Monday night, because the cafe was closed, and Ed was off work.

As their friendship developed, the couple told Ed how much he made them think of their own blue-eyed, blond-haired son, who would have been about Ed's age had he not died when he was a toddler. In appreciation for their friendship and home-cooked meals, Ed began showing up early on Mondays and found lots of work to do for them. He enjoyed making things look their best, he had the ability to see what needed to be done, and he had the energy to do it. The result was always attractive and orderly. Ed's handiwork was so appreciated by the old couple that they invited him to live at their ranch and work for them. They weren't in a position to pay him, but he would have a place to stay, a room of his own, and all the meals a growing young man could eat. The old man and Ed were about the same size, and he gave Ed some sturdy work jeans and several brightly colored cowboy shirts. At first Ed felt funny dressing like a cowboy, but he soon developed a liking for the bright colors and the feel of the jeans. He gladly exchanged them for his black clothing, which seemed to represent the dark past as opposed to the bright future he was creating for himself. He wanted to develop his skills and hobbies, and he had time in the evening to read. In exchange for all the work he was doing, he was encouraged to borrow the couple's old car to go to the town library and check out all the books he wanted.

The Law of Attraction had drawn these people together. For the first time Ed had a family who wanted him, took loving care of him, and urged him on his path of growth. He lived in a home that was warm and brightly lit, and shared it with people who genuinely cared about him. In return for their many kindnesses, they had the friendship of a delightful young man who was about the age of the son they had lost.

The Oregon ranch was small in size but big in projects. The long hours of each day were filled with labor, which built a strong, handsome body for Ed as the ranch took on a rustic beauty of its own. After supper, the three of them listened to country music on the radio with their big, yellow dog curled up by the fire. The couple would talk about such things as the Great Depression and evolution. The old man would play the guitar, and Ed added playing the guitar to his love of reading. With so many things fixed and working better than they ever had before, Ed had time to turn his attention to the couple's horse. He had never been around horses, and, although initially he was intimidated, he eventually befriended the horse and won her acceptance. Finding an old saddle in the barn and using the guidelines from a library book, he learned how to put on the tack and saddle the horse. One afternoon, after getting up his courage, he gingerly mounted the horse and made a loop around the corral. The Law of Attraction had just escorted Ed into a new era of his life.

Ed and that horse became inseparable. He rode her everywhere, and his desire to take the best care of her had him checking out every equestrian book on the library shelves. He learned about grooming, training, riding, feeding, and all other manner of horse care. He noticed how the horse's hooves looked different from those in the illustrations in his books, so he got a book on basic horse foot care and some tools from the feed store and barn, and he started to trim and reshape the horse's long-neglected hooves. She was patient with his efforts and probably felt his love for her, and before long she was showing off beautifully manicured hooves.

Having the interest and a growing belief in his ability to work with horses' hooves, Ed found a correspondence course for farriers. After many lessons, he earned his certificate in farriering and became a local horseshoer. His gentle spirit, good looks, and go-getter attitude won him the respect of ranchers throughout the county. Before long, he was shoeing horses far and wide, and making a good income doing it.

Ed had been with the couple for about 18 months when the old woman's younger sister and her daughter, who were down on their luck, came to visit. They arrived expecting to find the old couple in poor health and the ranch dilapidated. Much to their surprise, conditions were just the opposite. Things were in such good shape that they decided to move in and live there. As the relatives were moving in, Ed could see how important it was to the old couple to have their family there to take care of them. He knew that his time there was ending. He had had a meaningful and nourishing time, and now it was time to move on to attract the next chapter in his life—and attract he would, because he was clear about what he wanted: to stay out of trouble, to make wherever he was the best it could be, and to create the best life possible.

Knowing that his adopted family was in good hands, he said goodbye to the horse, the cow, the old, yellow dog, and the old couple who'd meant so much to him and from whom he had learned so much about how living together like a family could be. After a farewell breakfast at the cafe where it had all started, the couple put Ed, his farrier tools, his guitar, and his duffle bag full of bright-colored clothes on a southbound bus.

Ed's subsequent adventures took him on an odyssey of ranches, rodeos, carnivals, prairies, mountains, and farms. His boyish good looks, strong build, willingness to work, winning smile, and bright blue eyes always guaranteed him a job, friendship, and hospitality. It seemed as though he was living a charmed life.

Ed worked his way through the mountains of Montana and the horse ranches of Oregon and Washington. He traveled with a carnival and competed on a rodeo circuit while tending to horses and their feet along the way. Eventually he found work in California at a dude ranch as a wrangler. He shod the horses and mules, and escorted vacationing families to their campsites for memorable family outings. He freshened up the camp and cooked dinner, and afterward he and the guests sat around the fire while Ed played his old guitar, singing cowboy songs and amazing them with cowboy stories. In return, the vacationers rewarded him with gratuities, but most of all they treated him with respect and appreciation.

Ed was working at a ranch in the valley of the Owens River near Bishop, California, when a petite blonde named Gayle came into the rental office and asked if someone could help tack up her horse. Ed was immediately infatuated with the person who he later described as "the cutest little thing" he'd ever seen. After he tacked up her horse, she rode off, and Ed was summoned to run an errand into town. When he returned, Gayle had put her horse in its stall and was gone. There didn't seem to be any way to find her, and Ed felt a big emptiness. A few weeks later, friends invited him to dinner. When he arrived, much to his delight, he found that the woman they had told him they wanted him to meet was Gayle! After dinner Ed sang and spun yarn after yarn, infatuating his listeners and melting Gayle's heart. The Law of Attraction had brought the cowboy his own cowgirl, and it brought Gayle the promise of a future filled with love, companionship, and commitment, which were just the things she needed, because she was recovering from a history of bad relationships.

Ed and Gayle were married at a dude ranch in sunny Palm Springs, California, the following summer. I had had the privilege of meeting Ed while I was on a *City Slickers*–inspired cattle drive with my wife. Hearing his stories, I could tell that a part of the richness of his character had been developed while he managed his life and circumstances and pulled himself up by his bootstraps. One of my favorite memories is sitting on a horse facing Ed and Gayle, who were also on horseback, and officiating as the minister for their wedding. As the ceremony began at a dude ranch in Palm Springs, California, Gayle rode a beautiful horse to the appointed ceremony site. The guests admired her white wedding gown, which was draped over the horse's rump. The tiny sparkles on it and in her veil shimmered in the afternoon light. She looked radiant. The music of Purcell's "Trumpet Voluntary" floated in the air amid the sparkles. Suddenly there was a loud "Yea Hoo!" in the distance that drew everyone's attention to a cloud of dust and a tuxedoed cowboy thundering down the hillside on a horse that was going full-speed ahead. It was Ed!

Reading Ed's story, you can see that he followed the formula, and the Law of Attraction couldn't resist coming to his aid. After you accept this concept of empowering your life with thinking and creating, your next step is to accept delivery of your catalog of possibilities and beliefs. It will be delivered to you in many ways: perhaps while you're watching television, while you are talking to a friend, or during a challenging time. Once it arrives, take time to peruse the possibilities. Then decide what you want, be prepared to take action, and go to work.

Your Map to "I'll Accept Delivery of My Catalog of Possibilities and Beliefs"

Let empowered thinking and creativity stimulate the Law of Attraction.

Start anticipating the delivery of your catalog of possibilities and beliefs.

Expect to receive powerful visions of what you have the power to manifest.

Once your catalog has arrived, peruse it and start making a list of the possible projects inviting themselves into your life.

Enjoy the process of attracting your possibilities as you watch them present themselves to you.

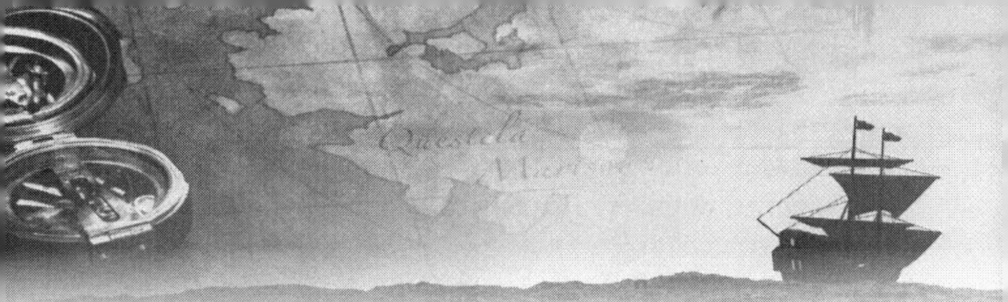

Chapter 5

What Do You Want?

The strongest principle of growth lies in human choice.

~ George Eliot (1891–1880), novelist

LET'S review what you've learned and hopefully accomplished thus far in your journey of creating the life you desire. You've developed a greater consciousness of how powerful your thoughts are to bring about a new, more productive awareness. You have an increased sense of how creative you are to manifest these results. And, hopefully, you see that with the motivation to set new goals and experience dynamic results in your life, you will activate the Law of Attraction, which will deliver your own catalog of possibilities and beliefs. Now you're ready to decide what you want and claim it.

Put another way, it's time to ask: "What do I want?" This question is also helpful when dealing with others, especially when they're upset or angry. Asking them "What do you want?" is like asking "What will fix the problem?" You can get to the solution quickly and avoid hearing all the details of what went wrong. Not only does this work with others, but it's a tool you can use to help yourself. With this question in mind, you'll avoid having to go through all the details and excuses of what went wrong, who hurt you, how this always happens, and so forth, if you simply say, "Yeah, yeah, I know all that, but what do I want that I don't have?"

Here's my list of some of the things people want.

The most important thing on everyone's list is results. Results come in the form of gratification, satisfaction, happiness, feelings of success, recognition, and income.

Second, people long for a sense of purpose and a destination that will be fulfilling. We all want to see results, and we want to see them quickly. However, people think they can't have what they want because too many obstacles stand in their way. Maybe these perceived obstacles keep them from learning how to be a ballroom dancer, or a guitar player, or a karaoke singer. The truth is, however, that each of these barriers can be overcome with determination.

> *If you limit your choices only to what seems possible or reasonable, you disconnect yourself from what you truly want, and all that is left is a compromise.*
>
> ~ Robert Fritz (b. 1943), management consultant

You *can* have what you want. The only thing that's stopping you is your limited thinking. For instance, let's say you desire to become an astronaut who wears a spacesuit and soars through the galaxies. But you've had too many birthdays, and there isn't enough time for you to get the education and the flight training required for such a position. Your feeling of defeat and not being able to reach your desired goal can disable you. The next thing you know, you're living life as a failed person instead of being the successful person you're meant to be.

Let's take this imagined story further. You realize what you're doing to yourself by thinking "I can't have what I want," and you change the story you're telling yourself. Now you say, "I can think and create a way to have what I want or something better." Then you go to the local aerospace museum and volunteer to be a docent. You gain self-respect as you inspire the young students whose school trips brought them to the museum. Your passion for what you teach is so contagious that the powers that be promote you to a senior position. You come up with the idea of making your presentations about space exploration wearing one of the museum's official spacesuits while sitting in the space capsule on exhibit.

Look at what you've created: You wear a spacesuit, you sit in a capsule, and you and your "crew"—the students—soar through the galaxies together, bringing you the respect and adoration of an audience that thinks you're terrific.

But, the greatest prize of all is that you overcame the negative thinking that said, "I can't have what I want." Hopefully this story will inspire you to take command and create what you want. My own inspiration was a grandmother who took tap dance lessons at the senior center. She was a natural at it, and she awakened a long-hidden dream to be performing on stage. At first, it seemed as though too many birthdays were holding her back from this lifelong vision. Besides, she reasoned, who wanted to watch an old woman tap dance?

She was inspired to volunteer at a local dance studio, where she had an audience that loved her and whom she could teach. These eager little dancers not only learned how to dance and perform, but they also learned about overcoming barriers that can hold back success and how to break through them.

Once you master the belief that you can have what you want and are aware that how it manifests itself might be different from how you first envisioned it, you're on your way.

One of my favorite affirmations is "If it is to be, it is up to me." Claiming responsibility and being willing to do the work and take the time (being patient along the way) will bring you the desired results or something better. Go ahead and think in terms of something better, because the results will look better on the other side of the finish line than they do from the starting line.

Remember: The results you desire are built by you. You are your own programmer. Using your conscious mind, you can create order, you can become focused, you can develop consciousness, and you can formulate a map to your desired destination. You can and must become motivated and ready to take action.

To have what you want, it's your responsibility to decide what input you wish to accept. This input might be coming from family history, a lack of belief in yourself, a track record of failed beginnings, or other negative sources. You are the master programmer here. Find the delete button and push it, making way for input that will support your progress and not interrupt it. Remember: Our greatest allies are interest, consciousness, inner locus of control, focus, and action. What you focus on consistently will find its way into your life. It's empowering to know that you created your results instead of thinking that they were created by fate or luck.

You can enjoy this power, because you have the ability to create what you desire. You can create a caring and supportive disposition. Your beliefs create the pattern by which your efforts bring results. What you hold in mind (focused, believing, and interested) constantly and persistently will take root and attach itself to you. Every deep-seated conviction, expectation, and emotion *will* translate into tangible results. Your thoughts and emotions determine your physical health, your life experience, and your ability to make changes in your life.

This process is similar to preparing a gourmet meal. Your first step is to develop an attitude of complete responsibility for the outcome of this project. If a wonderful meal is to be created, it will be because you'll see to it that it happens. You'll be responsible for the time it takes, as well as the cost and the results. You don't expect anyone else to do it for you or to rescue you if you have difficulty.

The second step is to decide what you want this project to accomplish. Perhaps your goal is the expression of friendship or love to your guests or the celebration of a success. You implement the third step as you put your goals in writing and visualize the results. You might see a beautifully set table with crystal and candlelight, or a charming country-style table with plaid napkins and fresh flowers. You might visualize the glow of pleasure on your friends' faces when they smell the delicious aroma of your meal. You play with your dreams in this phase of the process.

Now, you are ready to put your vision into action. You can create a time schedule of what you need to do. With paper and pencil, you create a specific menu, organize a guest list, select a date, put together a shopping list, and set in motion the process of making your desire a reality. The natural flow of creativity, coupled with your reasons for having the dinner, will come to your assistance. The results you've visualized and envisioned will take shape, and your dinner will be the result.

Develop an Attitude of Complete Responsibility for Your Life

The same process applies to the major challenges in life. Let's imagine that your goal is to have a healthy love relationship. You begin by knowing that healthy, loving relationships don't come about by accident. Without condemning, blaming, or judging others, take responsibility for the kind of relationships you've created in the past. Then take responsibility for creating the quality of relationships you want in the future.

Do you want to make an existing relationship more romantic, loving, and harmonious? Do you want to develop a committed relationship with someone you haven't met yet? Do you want to develop a circle of supportive friends? Do you want to improve your relationship with a child or a coworker? Be specific about exactly what you want to accomplish.

Develop a vision of how your relationships will be. Perhaps you envision a partner with whom you enjoy daily activities. For example, you might see your special person and you walking hand in hand. Perhaps your vision includes a picnic in a meadow or evenings of interesting conversation. Once you visualize your goal, put it in writing so you can focus on how to accomplish it.

Then develop a plan of action. What do you need to do to accomplish this goal? Let's imagine that you want to move your marriage from a state of bitterness and resentment to one of love and harmony. You might begin by working on your qualities of compassion and forgiveness. Decide on specific changes in your own behavior that will support your spouse so he or she can behave better toward you. Invest in spiritual or psychological counseling to help implement your changes. Write down your plan of action, set a time frame, and constantly keep your vision in focus.

Decide Exactly What You Want

How does one decide what he or she wants in life? We start by dividing our wants into specific areas. In general, these areas are relationships, health, and prosperity.

People often fail to clearly think through what they want in these areas. On the other hand, when we're inconvenienced by situations that frustrate us, we're able to observe what's desirable and undesirable. With this in mind, and with pen and paper in hand, make a list of what you'd like to have in each of these areas. Although your list can include generalities, specifics will draw you closer to deciding what you want. Look at what you can do to expand your accomplishments as well as how to minimize or eliminate what you don't like.

Another technique for discovering what you truly want is to pretend you have a magic wand. If you had such a wand and could make a wish, knowing that the wish would come true, what would you wish? An important creative concept to develop is one of making contact with an end result and holding it in your vision until it actualizes as a reality. The "in-between" stuff will be easier to focus on if you concentrate on the completed vision.

"But how do I get these things?" you might be asking. This kind of thinking has killed many happy endings. Be on your guard, and don't allow the in-between to cloud your ability to decide.

> *The words "I am..." are potent words; be careful what you hitch them to. The thing you're claiming has a way of reaching back and claiming you.*
>
> ~ A.L. Kitselman, motivational author

Grasping your magic wand firmly in your mind, ask such questions as these: "What would I really like to have in this area of my life? If I were unlimited in every way (intelligence, prosperity, education, ability), how would I think about my options to have all I want? How do I want to feel in this area? What do I expect to gain in having all I want? What would add to the quality of my life and look like success when I've gained it? What would I give back to the world, or a charity, or my family, to show my appreciation when I accomplish this goal?"

The contribution you make with your life can make a difference to the rest of us. The greater the quality of the contribution, the greater the quality of the difference. While one person might make a significant scientific discovery, another might write a symphony, and another might create a literary masterpiece. Each accomplishment serves to nurture and support each of us on our quest to discover what we want to achieve in our lives. While it might not be realistic for you to write a symphony, the inspiration of those who have done so is still there to help you express your own uniqueness in areas of your life that are just as important to your fulfillment as the composer's accomplishment is to him or her.

Remember that the time and energy you put into your decision is quality time. You're investing in your happiness and success. Through this process, you're likely to confront many of the robbers who can steal away your energy and conviction. You have the power to stir up the creativity and energy you'll need for the next step: adding animation to your written decision so it becomes vision.

A review of the ways to decide what you want includes the following:

Make a list of qualities you desire in the areas of relationships, health, and prosperity.

Use your magic wand, and let your imagination go. This is the way great ideas are formed.

Remain focused on the result so excuses and self-limiting thoughts don't interfere with your vision.

Remember that your success is proof that all things are possible and that we have the power to be all we envision ourselves to be.

A Case History in Deciding What You Want: Vicki's Story

The time was 1915. At age 15, Vicki had a pretty face, the body of a woman, and the heart of a dreamer, but she lived in a dreary, dusty, East Texas town called Gilmer. Her life consisted of going to school and doing farm chores and housework. Although she had siblings, the most difficult chores were assigned to her. Her parents were limited and often abusive. Vicki's only entertainment was to go to the lone drugstore in town, have a Coca-Cola at the fountain, and look at the movie magazines. Reading about the movie stars and their glamorous lives in faraway Hollywood gave her the stamina to live in her dreary town. She yearned for a life filled with glamour, wealth, and romance, which the pictures in the movie magazines seemed to reflect.

One day, while preparing to return to her meager home, Vicki stood on the drugstore's dusty, wooden porch. As her thoughts turned toward going to an unhappy home, she longed for something better. This dismal moment was interrupted when a black, open-topped touring car with headlights as big as dinner plates pulled up in front of her. It astonished Vicki to see a woman driving the car, and it astonished her further that the car was occupied by four or five other women.

The doors flew open, and the women emerged. Vicki had never seen women like these before. They were dressed in bright clothing with high-heeled shoes, and all of them wore nail polish and lip rouge. They were the closest thing to glamour that she had ever seen in Gilmer outside the movie magazines.

As the group passed Vicki on the porch, the driver of the car said, "Well, hi, darlin'. You're a pretty little thing. With a little fixin' up, you could be real pretty, darlin'."

Eventually, Vicki managed to ask, "What do you all do?"

One of them replied, "Oh, honey, we work in the oil fields."

Their quiet laughter was interrupted by Vicki's next question: "Do you drill for oil?"

The reply came back: "Oh, yes, honey. We drill!"

The wheels were turning in the mind of the woman who had been driving the car. She asked, "Honey, how old are you?"

Vicki replied, "I'm 15, but I'll be 16 in July."

"Do you live around here?"

Vicki replied yes, and the woman said, "Honey, why don't you come with us? We need a maid, and I think you'd do just fine."

Leave Gilmer, and have a life filled with travel, adventure, and pretty clothes? That sounded wonderful to Vicki! But her dreamy state was interrupted by a thought, and she said, "Oh, I can't go with you. My mama—"

"Oh, honey, your old mama would want you to go with us. Come along and go with us. We'll write your mama a letter and tell her you're okay, and we'll send her some money."

Vicki knew she should go home, but the idea of returning to what awaited her there seemed to help her leap into the car with the painted ladies and speed off into a life that promised adventure and beautiful things. She worked as a maid for these women, who drove from oil camp to oil camp entertaining and satisfying the needs of the lonely men who worked there. At some point, she was promoted from maid to being one of the girls. Although she knew that her choice wouldn't be approved back home, the glamour outweighed what she had heard in church.

Vicki's adventures took her to the "happening" city of Dallas. She worked hard practicing using makeup and arranging her hair to get that glamour look of the movie stars, and this put her in even higher demand with her gentlemen friends. She was escorted to some of Dallas's finest restaurants, nightclubs, theaters, and even the opera once. Heads turned when this dark-haired beauty walked into a room, often draped over the arm of some balding, boot-wearing oil millionaire who was out for a good time in the big city.

As fate would have it, she attracted the attention of a handsome young gambler named A.Z. Stephens. A.Z.'s brother was a traveling salesman for the Acme Boot Company. A.Z.'s occupation was to pull his shiny roadster full of empty boot boxes into a naïve Texas town, go to the local saloon, and tell everyone he was a boot salesman and that he hoped to get in a game of cards that evening. When evening came, he'd flash a big roll of money and lose miserably, with the promise to come back the next night and try his luck again. On the second night, aided by his deck of marked cards, he'd make a killing, scoop up the money, and excuse himself to the restroom with the promise of returning for more play. Instead, he'd slip out the restroom window and vanish before his cards were discovered, and then speed back to Dallas and into Vicki's arms.

Their life together took a curve when one of A.Z.'s gambling trips took him to Oklahoma, and he invited Vicki along. Their joyride in his fancy sports car was interrupted by a police car's siren. One of the lawmen asked A.Z. and Vicki where they were going. When the reply was "Oh, just out for a drive," the officer asked, "Are you aware that you're in Oklahoma? And are you aware of the Mann Act, which says it's against the law to bring women of questionable reputation across a state line?" The quick-thinking A.Z. said, "Oh, we've come to Oklahoma to get married," and the officer said, "Well, congratulations. Why don't you just follow me and we'll go just down the road a piece to a judge who can marry you today?"

Knowing the consequences of not following, A.Z. and Vicki followed him to the judge's office and were married on the spot. This was fine with both of them, but after a few months their passion cooled. When Vicki became pregnant, they tried to stay together, but after the baby was born, a girl they named Lou Nell, they broke up. A struggle ensued for custody. Using his influence (and perhaps a little cash), A.Z. had Vicki declared an unfit mother, and he gained custody. Then he gave Lou Nell to his sister Mary to raise in Austin, Texas. For Mary, this was an answered prayer; she and her husband had always wanted a child but could never have one.

Meanwhile in Dallas, Vicki went back to her glamorous life and work, but her adventures and trials with A.Z. had damaged her esteem—the way others saw her and the way she saw herself. Younger and more vivacious girls were being invited to be escorts. She also developed a tremendous health challenge: a cantaloupe-sized thyroid gland. Surgery was followed by a long recovery, during which Vicki couldn't work. During her recuperation, she found that she had time to read and acquire knowledge that she had always wanted but had never had the time to seek.

Using some of her savings, Vicki settled into a quiet life. Because her room in the rooming house was tiny, she sometimes read in the waffle shop nearby. It was there that she met a nice-looking, lonely, and very successful accountant. One day he offered to buy her lunch, their acquaintance became friendship, and that opened a door for them both. The accountant knew nothing about Vicki's background and was too naïve to figure it out, but he realized that he couldn't do without this woman. One day, he presented a large diamond engagement ring and proposed. Vicki realized that it would be best for her to retire from her previous profession and become his wife.

His accounting firm afforded them a quite comfortable level of living, and Vicki was soon attending operas, balls, cotillions, and church as the wife of a successful businessman. No one knew her past, but everyone reacted to her mature beauty and treated her respectfully, impressed by her "unsinkable Molly Brown" personality and style. She occasionally ran into one of her old gentlemen friends at a social event, but by silent agreement, they acted as though that was their first meeting.

After several years of this stable life, Vicki's husband died, leaving her a substantial estate, including their mansion in Highland Park, an exclusive Dallas neighborhood. As this next chapter of her life began, Vicki found herself involved in society and a member of the local Christian Science church with the reputation of being an outstanding volunteer. It was at this time that 18-year-old Lou Nell decided to visit her birth mother. It turned out to be a wonderful experience for mother and daughter, because by then Vicki was mature enough to foster a meaningful relationship. After many hours of their getting to know each other, Lou Nell decided to move to Dallas. She moved in with her mother and attended secretarial school and, on her frequent visits with Mary in Austin, she assured Mary that Vicki wasn't the evil person that Mary had been led to believe.

Eventually Lou Nell got a job as the coffee shop's cashier at the Adolphus Hotel in Dallas. There she met a handsome, hardworking bellhop named Art. They fell in love, married, and eventually had three children. Celebrating family occasions filled in a large gap in Vicki's life.

Vicki had come a long way from that day when she had stood on that boardwalk outside the drugstore in Gilmer to living in the mansion in Dallas, and her story perfectly illustrates the concepts you're learning about in our journey. Vicki reinvented herself several times, with images for herself and her life so clear that they activated the Law of Magnetism, and she became a society lady whose efforts raised vast amounts of money for charities and social service. Some people could say, "Yes, but look at what she did to get there," but Vicki's decision to have what she longed for—followed up with dreams and the clear vision of living a life of glamour—got her to her goal, and along the way she put herself in positions to gain character as attractive as her beauty.

Vicki's life is proof that when people have dreams and goals, and maintain the vision to reach them, they put themselves in the position to have adventures that outside observers can label good or bad, but these adventures can also add character and quality. If Vicki hadn't had the dreams, hadn't stepped into that touring car, and hadn't fallen in love with A.Z. and given birth to Lou Nell, I wouldn't be writing this book. I wouldn't even be here. This is because Lou Nell and Art were my mother and father, and Vicki was my grandmother.

Vicki's story illustrates something important to you as well:

You never know what deciding what you want, dreaming the dream, visualizing the goal, and letting the Laws of Attraction and Magnetism work in your life will bring. These things could bring circumstances that might be questionable from the outside, but dreaming, goal setting, and moving forward to accomplishment will activate the Law of Magnetism in bringing your goals to fruition.

Your Map to "I'll Attract My Catalog, Review My Options, and Decide What I Want"

Vicki's story contains your map to this island. Knowing that you can create the results you desire, let's look at the formula. There are three steps:

Develop an attitude of complete responsibility for your life.
Decide exactly what you want.
Be aware that the next step is to make sure you have the interest and belief that you can have what you want. Then you'll be prepared to put your goals in writing and develop the capacity to visualize the result and create a schedule for what you need to do.

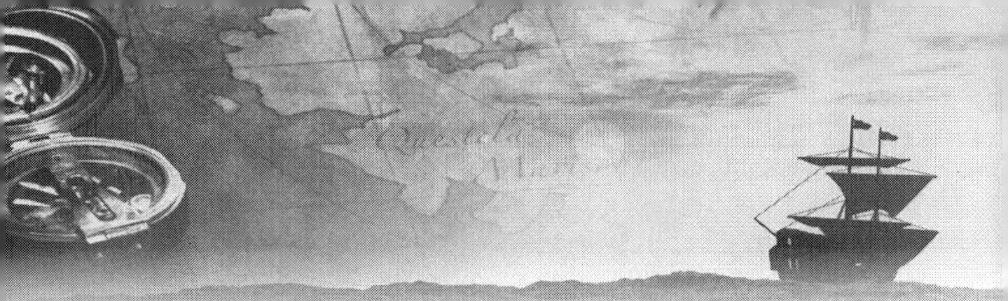

Chapter 6

Do You Have the Necessary Interest and Belief?

One thing life has taught me: if you are interested, you never have to look for new interests. They come to you. When you are genuinely interested in one thing, it will always lead to something else.

~ Eleanor Roosevelt (1884–1962),
first lady, columnist, and diplomat

REMEMBER that sea monster in Chapter 1? In this chapter, we'll be doing some serious monster slaying. The two sea monsters that must be overcome are Lack of Interest and Lack of Belief. The excitement and fun begin once you have harnessed your understanding of how powerful your thoughts are and how creative you can be. Then, this awareness of your powers of thought and creativity starts stimulating your ability to attract an awareness of all the possibilities that are your reward for slaying these two monsters. The next thing you know, you start to visualize results that are created by diligent work and application, and you realize that you're on your journey to the most productive life you've ever experienced.

You really can feel like an explorer headed for a great

conquest. You leave the Harbor of Thought and sail to the "I'll Create," where you receive your first welcome. While your ship and crew (talents and abilities) are still fresh and energetic, you set sail for "I'll Receive," where your catalog of possibilities and beliefs is delivered. And while you peruse its many possibilities, you realize that this trip isn't as scary as you originally thought but that it is truly an adventure, and you're having fun. Then you set sail for your next port. On the way you encounter the two sea monsters, Lack of Interest and Lack of Belief, and realize that it's you or them. Having invested so much of yourself and having come this far, you must make the decision to eliminate these two monsters if you're going to return home with all the promised rewards.

Let's look at some ways to turn these foes into friends. I have an exercise I do in some of my seminars that might create as big a breakthrough for you as it has for my participants. First, I ask the people in my audience to relax, close their eyes, take a few deep breaths, and then imagine a wild beast just a few feet in front of them. As I'm watching them, I see many of them immediately tighten up and their posture change from relaxed to tense. Their faces show anxiety, and they act uneasy. Then I tell them to look closely at the ferocious beast so they can describe its appearance. Then I ask them to be prepared to explain how they react to it. Finally, I ask them to open their eyes and give me feedback about their experience.

The most vivid descriptions I get are from those people with the best imaginations. They report big, hairy, snarling, drooling beasts, fire-breathing dragons several stories tall, wooly mammoths with pointed tusks, and so on. (Once, a man reported his ferocious beast to be his mother-in-law.)

When I ask them to explain what they do in reaction to the monster they've created, the answer is consistently the same: They run for their lives!

At this point in my experiment I ask them to close their eyes, get comfortable, and go back to the scene where they last saw their monster. I assure them that they won't get hurt. Then I ask them to see the monster just as it was before, snarling and ready to do what they thought it was going to do at the time of their last visit. Then I ask them to freeze the scene and be prepared to identify a powerful idea. Then I say, "This monster is your monster. You created it out of your imagination. It only has the power you give it. You made it ferocious and scary, and now it has you running for your life. You have surrendered your power to something you have imagined. You can take the power you gave it back, tame the monster, and make it work for your benefit."

Then I ask the people in my audience to unfreeze their monster and turn it into a creature as tame and playful as a puppy. I invite them to keep it its original size, and then to put a leash on it and take it for a walk. Now they're in charge of something that just moments earlier had them running for cover. Then I ask them to open their eyes and tell me where they went on their walk. The reports are amazing. People in my seminars have taken their monsters home to show their kids or to work, where they breathed fire and shook things up. One imaginative person took his monster to Hollywood, where it became a famous horror film star, made a monstrous salary, and lived in a huge Beverly Hills estate.

If I Hadn't Believed It

> *The thing always happens that you really believe in: and the belief in a thing makes it happen.*
>
> ~ Frank Lloyd Wright (1867–1959),
> architect and interior designer

A friend of ours recently made a statement that sounded as if it might have come from Frank Lloyd Wright: "If I hadn't believed it, I wouldn't have seen it." There was a truth hidden in that statement. "If I hadn't believed it, I wouldn't have seen it" means it's not that you see something and then you believe it, but that you believe it and then it appears.

Good ways to think about this concept are: "As I believe it, I achieve it," and "As I believe it, I see it." Often, "the way it is" is not the way it is, but the way I believe it to be. When I can believe that something can be better, then I will see it, because I believed it.

All we really need to do, then, is go to that place in our mind where we do our thinking and ask: "What do I believe about this situation? What have I been told about this situation? What are the clichés I've collected along the way? What do I want to see? What do I think and how do I feel? What are my expectations, and where am I going?" And, "In my collection of thoughts, which ones are limiting me and holding me back from creating what I desire?"

Taking this approach will pinpoint where you are, and you'll be able to see how far you've come. You'll be able to increase your understanding of the power that you have. As you increase this awareness, the frustrations, anxieties, and problems will decrease so everything becomes manageable.

And then, understanding yourself, you can look at your beliefs and envision results through belief. As you see those achievements in your vision of the future, you'll eventually be able create tangible results. Whatever you establish as a goal has to first be believed. Then you can say, "If I hadn't believed it, I wouldn't have seen it."

Giving all your attention to the negative and ignoring the positive causes the negative to expand. I knew a woman who appeared to have it all. She had a husband who loved her, great kids, the lovely house she'd always dreamed of having, and great parents. In spite of this, she chose to dwell on the negative. This woman was concerned about how stuck she thought she was in her situation. She was driving down the freeway one day, focusing on what was wrong in her life, when another driver lost control of his car and sandwiched the woman between the guardrail and the other car. She said later, "You really start having some creative ideas when the sparks from the guardrail are going past your window, and it looks like you're in a fireworks show with a bridge coming up for the finale."

When everything stopped and she was able to get out of her car, she realized that she could have been killed. She knew she had been giving too much time and energy to negative thinking and needed to change, but she didn't do it until she was, in her words, "blasted up to the next level."

I think of life as a spiral staircase. We are on one step for a while, learning all that step in life has to offer, and, when we've completed our mission there, we take the next step up. You can tell when it's time to take that next step when the one you're on feels old and used up. At this point, you choose to move up to the next step, you decide what you want, you believe there's something better waiting for you, and you follow your dreams and grow out and grow up. If we don't choose to grow when life offers us the advances, we're "blasted up" to the next level.

I can vividly remember times in my life when I've been blasted up to a new level of responsibility and productivity. I created my own blast by failing to choose to follow the calling to climb higher. Either way, by choice or by blast, the importance of reaching new levels of life applies to all of us. As for my above-mentioned friend, all heaven broke loose—and some hell, too, which caused her to realize that she had outgrown the level she was on, where all she focused on was the negative. She stepped up to a higher level of living and began to be more thankful.

If you choose to grow, life offers you the advances as if all heaven breaks loose—and some hell, too. We all reach those times when we're up against the wall. To prevent ourselves from being blasted up to the next level, and moving up by choice, each of us needs to have a meeting in the boardroom of our minds. You're the executive director. You are the president of You, Incorporated. You're the president of the board, with the ability to ratify or veto everything that happens. Sometimes you might have to say, "I don't remember ratifying that; I don't remember approving this." Some things happen that you could have vetoed if you had been thinking and being the responsible individual you know yourself to be.

Hold a Board Meeting in Your Mind

Let's have a board meeting in your mind. In this citadel of power and love, there's an upper room that has a big conference table. You sit at the head of the table, and the members of your board (your faculties) are all gathered around. All the things that are right about you and all the things that are wrong about you are there.

When you enter your boardroom, take your place at the head of the table, close your eyes, place your feet flat on the floor to bring up the energy, and open your hands to receive. In this position of openness and reflection, you can think correctly. While you sit at the head of the table, all your faculties are on either side of you. All the power is present, mustered to help you get all the guidance you need.

You might begin by saying: "This is what I want." Then you might ask, "Does anyone have any advice?" Then, get ready for lots of reaction. You must realize that some of your reactions come from what you've been told to think by others. The patterns of thinking that have made the most impressions on us are from our parents, bosses, friends, and love relationships. It's critical to sort all that out, discarding negative beliefs that don't serve you and that even interfere with the results you want.

The people who raised and shaped you as best they could

taught you their beliefs about how the world works. From them, you learned patterns of thinking and expectations. You were also told about the members of your family who have always been clumsy, lazy, poor, rich, or forgetful. You can dwell on family history and old beliefs, or you can be free to go to your boardroom, call order, and develop a belief system that gives you power.

It is important not only to be a positive thinker but also a positive knower. This is easy to describe as positive thinking, but I like to think of it as positive believing. What you think is important, but what you know is what *is*. You might be thinking one thing and knowing something else. You might be thinking positively, yet you know it's going to be "one of those days." You are here to reform your thinking; life is a reform school. When you change your thinking to accommodate truths, the events in your life will fall into place in proper perspective.

At your board meeting, as you gather your thoughts, your inner voice might sound like this: "Now this is what I know: I would like more order in my life. I would like my surroundings to be more orderly or more beautiful or more conducive to the way I want to live. I want more happiness in my job and more up-to-date transportation. I want loving, significant relationships."

If you get what you ask for and find out it wasn't what you wanted, you can go back to your boardroom and try again. Doing this will keep you on track, so you can see the results that you're capable of creating as an assertive, responsible individual. You'll want to make these results your goals. When you know what you want, write it down. Don't forget the importance of placing your goals and desires in writing, and place them where you can see them every day.

Follow Your Board Meeting with Action!

Be not afraid of life. Believe that life is worth living, and your belief will help create the fact.

~ William James (1842–1910), psychologist and philosopher

When you know what you want and believe you're going to have it, the appropriate action becomes clear. Perhaps you want to create more order in your life. Maybe you need to clean up the mess in the garage and take the excess to the rummage sale or give it to the poor. Maybe you need to make everything brighter—paint and clean that shelf, and move things around so they don't look the same.

Knowing what you want and believing you can have it make you alert to opportunities. As you affirm your vision, you draw new opportunities to you and recognize what's already available. With your vision in mind, all you have to do is take action. When you know what you believe and what you want, some really incredible things will start to move in your world. People who discipline themselves in this manner are called movers and shakers. Their world moves and shakes because they go for the results they want. When you learn to discipline your thinking, you achieve peace of mind. You'll have the ability to bring all you need into your life. You'll have so much that you'll have to recycle everything.

Remember: It all comes from thought! As you take charge of your thinking and shift to positive thinking, positive feelings follow. These feelings will help you to be adaptive and appropriate in your action and behavior.

Do You Have the Interest?

For this to work you need to be genuinely interested in changing your thoughts. When I was considering the importance of interest, I recalled something that happened a while ago. In addition to giving keynote speeches, I present classes and seminars on wealth and prosperity. At the end of my presentations, I offer books and CDs that usually aren't purchased by the senior citizens in my audience. I was curious about why older people had no interest in taking home the information about prosperity. At the conclusion of some of my seminars, I asked a couple of the very senior citizens of my audience if they'd like a copy of the seminar. I explained that the CD was my gift to them. They consistently replied, "No, thank you." When I asked, "May I ask why you don't want my gift to you?" their answers went like this: "We are old, we live off our retirement, we aren't going back to work, and there's no way we can have more money."

It was evident that they didn't have an interest in wealth or increasing prosperity in their lives. I think this lack of interest was fostered by a belief that they couldn't have any more income or money than they had because they were on a limited income, they were retired, and they couldn't work. These mindsets were killing their power of thought. This kind of thinking was limiting these older people from living more prosperous lives.

What if they surrendered the way they think and really became interested in finding ways to increase their prosperity? What if they added positive belief to this formula?

Let's look at the ways they could increase their prosperity. They could use their life skills and volunteer someplace that, in return, would give them satisfaction money can't buy. They could become expert consultants and be paid for sharing their wealth of experience. They could write a book about the adventures they've had in life. The list goes on and on, and it starts with the power of thought. Many older people have wound up richer at the end of their lives than when they started because they were truly interested in increasing their personal wealth and believed that they could. Two who come to mind are Clara Peller (the "Where's the beef?" woman) and Grandma Moses. As you nurture interest, you will create new ways to think.

Are You an Owner or a Renter?

Our next step in creating thinking that makes you a winner is taken when you decide to be an owner instead of a renter. Let me explain. Recently I was hungry for an ice cream cone. I went inside an ice cream shop to find the single employee sitting on the counter talking on the phone. She didn't greet me or look in my direction. I could clearly hear her conversation, which was obviously not work-related. She was talking about a boy she knew and why he had broken up with her friend.

Her conversation went on for two or three minutes. Finally she said she had to go, and that she would call the friend back soon. Then she slid off the countertop and came over to me. Still not saying a word, she looked at me with that "So?" look that disinterested people often display. I asked for a chocolate ice cream cone. She said, "That will be a dollar fifty-six." I gave her two dollars, and she gave me my change. I said, "Thank you" and left the store. She never said "You're welcome" or "Good-bye" or "Come again, please." Although I got what I wanted, I didn't get prompt service, attention, or recognition, which are the things that bring a costumer back.

Using my power of thought, I put on my Sherlock Holmes hat and asked myself some questions. I wanted the outcome of my experience to be a pleasant one. I was interested in the way my interpretation of the experience would shape my feelings, and I believed I could search my thoughts and find something positive that I could use in my presentations.

I asked some questions and did some thinking that brought me to some conclusions. First, I didn't personalize the employee's behavior as directed at me personally. I realized that she probably treated every customer this way. Second, I realized that this person was probably not the owner of the shop. Third, it was clear that she saw herself as an employee. With further insight I discovered my own belief that "wannabe" owners often start out as employees who work diligently to promote themselves and their dream of being an owner someday.

My conclusion was that ownership is a decision. I think you either decide "I'm just an employee; I'll always be an employee; I'll never be an owner," or you decide "Someday I'm going to own this." A big principle in successful goal reaching is concentrating on the goal, not on how it will be accomplished. The "how" part will happen (with a lot of work and discipline) once the goal is established and is clearly in one's sight.

My final conclusion was that people can be employees, and if they work like they own the place, before long their efforts will attract positive attention, and they'll receive the promotions, increases in responsibilities, and income that they deserve. Their reputation with themselves and their peers will increase. Their behavior and beliefs will help them develop into owner material.

So let me ask: At your job, are you an owner, or are you just an employee? At home, and with your friends, are you just there, or do you own your place there?

When you make a decision to own your life, you'll create results that a mere employee can never enjoy. Own it! Remember: Your thoughts are your power. They are the blueprint upon which your life is built.

An Encounter with Patricia

Several months ago, knowing that I'd be writing a chapter that included the topic of interest and belief, I gave myself an assignment. I challenged myself to develop an interest in something with which I had little experience and that wouldn't ordinarily be of curiosity to me. I included developing an attitude of believing that I could follow through with this task. I decided to begin my search to find something that had been uninteresting that day, and the deadline was dusk. My wife and I enjoy skiing, and, during the morning, I searched the ski runs for a situation to meet my assignment and found nothing. Later, in the resort's dining room, what I was looking for found me before I knew what was happening.

The dining room is actually a chalet atop June Mountain at June Lake, California. It has a stunning view of the mountains that surround the lake and its village of shops, ski and boat rentals, restaurants, and inns. The room is usually full of skiers of all ages, circulating through its cafeteria line and dining tables like people at an after-Christmas sale. Children, parents, young snowboarders, and old skiers all want to grab some quick nourishment and get back on those slopes to get all the exercise and fun they can out of their expensive lift tickets. They're dressed in bulky, colorful clothes, with trays full of food, beverages, hats, and gloves. As soon as they find a table, they wolf down their lunch, and then they're off to the slopes. They're usually so eager to go play that they leave their cafeteria trays, dishes, glasses, and napkins behind.

While I was observing this scene and searching for something to find a new interest in, I noticed someone standing in front of me. As I looked up at her, I realized that I had seen her many times before but had never really noticed her. Her nametag said "Patricia." I realized that she was one of the people who worked on the mountain whose job it was to bus tables and clean up the messes the skiers left behind. Patricia was cheery, hardworking, and fast at clearing tables. I could see how hard she was working, but she seemed invisible and lost in the crowd of skiers. No one in the room seemed interested in her; they just saw her as someone who worked there. They didn't acknowledge her or thank her for doing the important job of keeping things clean and having table space cleared and ready for the next person.

Because she was working directly in front of me clearing someone else's mess, I spoke to her and said something like, "Hi, Patricia. You're really working hard today." She replied, "Yes, this job keeps me pretty busy," to which I said, "People surely can be messy, can't they?" She said, "Yep, but they're on vacation, and they're having fun."

At this point, I knew I had the subject matter for my self-imposed assignment, just as I'd believed I would. I asked Patricia, "So what's it like, working on the mountain?" Her reply was full of information. She explained that working on the mountain was a good job with "pretty good" pay and always a lot to do. The guests were interesting even if they were a bit messy. "But the real reason I love this job," she said, "is because as an employee, my kids get to ski for free."

My heart melted, and my appreciation for this seemingly invisible "just a bus person" went sky-high. I realized that she was doing what many would consider less-than-meaningful work so her children could ski. This helped them build healthy bodies and self-esteem, and gave them a productive place to be while their mother was at work. I was interested!

I continued my research in the days and lunchtimes that followed, and Patricia and I visited often. I came to see that behind the appearance of a seemingly invisible and unacknowledged worker was a special woman: a mother, an American

Indian from the Paiute tribe, an artist who made beautiful beaded jewelry, and, most of all, a person of substantial presence.

At the end of the ski season, I asked Patricia what she'd be doing during the summer. She explained that her children would be in summer school while she made jewelry and worked for the Bureau of Land Management. I knew the BLM as the organization that rounds up wild mustangs for adoption and for the protection of their species on the prairie. Upon further questioning, Patricia explained how she and several other American Indians would take large, plastic tubs and tennis rackets, and beat the local sage and berry bushes to collect seeds. Their collections would be bagged for the BLM, taken to burned or eroded land, and sprinkled on these areas. Then she explained how the deer would eat the seed, wrap it in fertilizer, and put it back on the ground, so when the rains came the seed would grow and replenish the land.

My quest to develop the qualities of interest and belief was a success. Looking back, I can see that its success came because I was genuinely interested, and I believed I could reach my learning goal and have material for this chapter of my book. In addition to proving my theory, I made a new friend. I'm glad to know Patricia and her family, and just think what I'd have missed if I had just seen her as an invisible individual who worked for the mountain at an unspectacular job. You can transform yourself as well if you are truly interested, and have a deep and abiding belief that you can reach your goal. You must also be willing to do the work, which will include developing the ability to take on new beliefs and ideas and create a new consciousness, clean house, focus on your desired results, become genuinely interested in the process, and keep on doing the work.

After accepting delivery of your catalog of possibilities and beliefs and becoming aware of what can be yours, it's important that you go deeply within and ask yourself these three questions: (1) Do I have genuine interest in pursuing and acquiring this goal? (2) Do I really believe I can do what needs to be done and have this result? (3) Am I willing to do the work this goal deserves?

As you take on the process of transforming yourself, you'll produce new thoughts, patterns, and feelings. These new areas of your consciousness will become reflected in your life, and you'll see results quickly. *Modeling* is a psychological term for imitating how one sees others and incorporates their actions and style into one's own way of doing what they do. You can model results in your life by seeing the results you want as a possibility, and by modeling you can affect your own life experience. I invite you to become a model and demonstrate your success for yourself and those around you. Perhaps as you reflect your expanded consciousness, you'll inspire other people, and they'll imitate you. This might just be the best way you could change the world.

Looking at other models might give you some new ideas to generate a change in your thinking. "Standing on the Shoulders of Giants" (Chapter 1) reminded us to be aware of how these giants must have had a keen sense of interest coupled with the belief that they could achieve the goal they desired and followed up by doing the work required. For instance, let's look at the lives of two princesses who were born into an agenda that dictated that someday they would be married off to sovereigns to expand kingdoms and perhaps eliminate devastating wars.

I've already told you about the German princess Catherine, who at age 15 was sent to Russia to be groomed to marry the future Russian emperor. The other giant, Princess Marie Antoinette, was sent at about the same age from Austria to France to be groomed to marry to the future king of France. By studying the results of their lives and the interest (or lack of interest) and the beliefs (or lack of beliefs) that they harbored, we can benefit from the work they did (or didn't do) in developing their own consciousness and their successes or failures.

Each was raised in court life and tutored on how to accommodate her husband. No expense was spared to expose them to court life, with its political intrigue, formalities, and practices.

Catherine took the future role she was born to execute quite seriously. She had the interest, and she believed that one day she would be in a position of power and influence. Thus, she made the most of her training and upbringing. Sure enough, her awareness resulted in a reign that changed the future of her adopted country and the rest of the world. Her incredible results, including the love and respect of her subjects, earned her the title of Catherine the Great.

The other princess, Marie Antoinette, didn't take the future role she was born to execute as seriously. Perhaps she hadn't developed an interest in being of service to her subjects. Surely she had the training and upbringing of a future monarch. But judging by her results, it's questionable that she had the interest it would take to pursue the role seriously that she was in line to perform. Her keenest interest appears to have been in pomp, circumstance, and the finery and luxury of palace life. She was more interested in a life of self-indulgence than in service to her country. Perhaps she never grasped the possibility of the contribution she could have made because she didn't have the genuine interest or the beliefs that such a significant future required. Marie Antoinette's lack of these two all-important qualities was so lacking that she lost her head.

Therein is the moral of these examples: Develop genuine interest and a deep belief that you can acquire the things and results you desire, and they (or something better) will be yours, or proceed toward your goals with aloof interest and a lack of belief that you can achieve your results, and you will lose your head.

Your Map to "I'll Develop Interest and Belief"

Develop and cultivate genuine interest in manifesting the things you want that appear in your catalog of possibilities.

Make sure you really believe these things can be yours and that you can accomplish whatever you set your mind and talents to creating.

Be prepared to do the work that will need to be done to stick to your commitment and to set goals that you will accomplish.

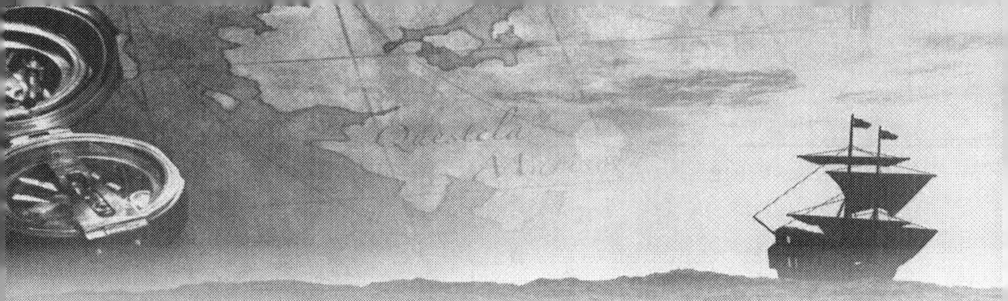

Chapter 7

Say Yes: Create Your Goals, and Put Them in Writing

A goal is a dream with a deadline.

~ Napoleon Hill (1883–1970),
motivational speaker and author

LET'S look at how far we've progressed on our journey of self-discovery. We developed an awareness that assures our success. Then we went to the "I'll Create" and discovered the power we have to take our best ideas and bring them to life. Our journey then took us to "I'll Attract," where we learned to put our thinking and creating to work to activate the Law of Attraction, which brought our catalog of possibilities and beliefs. Then we had to face the two sea monsters: Lack of Interest and Lack of Belief. Once we disciplined these monsters, they turned into aids for our campaign to venture into the unknown, discover vast treasures, and return to our homeport (thinking) to display our catch, collect our rewards, and embark on many other conquests.

We've accomplished a lot of the important groundwork necessary for the fun part of our journey. Now that we've overcome the Lack of Interest and Lack of Belief, it's time to go back to our catalog of possibilities, put in our order, and claim what is ours to create. It's time to put our goals in writing and develop the capacity to visualize the results.

This step in getting what you want is the most important and possibly the most difficult. Making it through this process is almost a guarantee of success, because developing a purpose or mission statement and visualizing what you want as yours is the starting point for real results.

> *By recording your dreams and goals on paper, you set into motion the process of becoming the person you most want to be. Put your future in good hands: your own.*
>
> ~ Mark Victor Hansen (b. 1948),
> inspirational speaker and author

Goals must be put in writing so we can be specific in our focus about what we want. When we think of our goals, we are often too general and non-specific. For instance, Sears and Roebuck (I don't know what happened to Roebuck) is famous for catalog sales. If you desired something from Sears, you wouldn't call the order department and say, "Send me something." You'd tell the sales rep that you'd like a specific item, found on page number so-and-so, and give the color and the size. Then you would provide your address and credit card info. In order to get what you want, you would have to be very specific.

What we want for ourselves can be attained in steps. Starting is often the challenge, and a substantial start seems to perpetuate itself through each step. Therefore, the time and effort you put into this step will have many positive payoffs. You might start out with a volume of needs and reduce it to the size of a chapter, then refine it to paragraphs, and then fine-tune it into a sentence or two. This process of deciding what you want will fine-tune not only your goals but also your ability to reach them. The most popular areas for goal setting are spiritual goals (getting closer to God), relationship goals (having a loving marriage), physical goals (losing weight), emotional goals (becoming calmer), career goals (becoming a manager), creativity goals (writing a book or song), and financial goals (having enough money to buy that dream house).

Having your goals in written form and having given thought and imagination to them while writing them will produce a chart to help you stay on course and reach the result you desire. Each written goal will become your mission statement and should be placed in your home or office, where you'll come in contact with it several times each day. In this way, you can be reminded of what you desire and can check your moment-to-moment progress. Many people find it equally helpful to keep their goal or mission statement in their pocket or purse, where they can read it several times during the day. I like to keep a copy of my goals in the shirt pocket over my heart. After all, they are my heart's desire. Others say that rewriting their goals each day refreshes not only their mind but also their capabilities.

You might look as this phase of your journey as your new job. The harder you work at it, the more likely that opportunity will take notice of your determination and reward you with results. By doing all you can to keep your goals on the tip of your mind, you'll also activate the Law of Magnetism, which we will discuss in an upcoming chapter.

Hopefully by now, you have been motivated to follow through with this step and put your goals in writing. These written goals are for your eyes only, and your first draft might ramble, but the clearer you are in determining what you want, the more specific you can become. Because this is your private copy of your goals, you can edit it and add whatever language is clear and deliberate to keep you on track. Be specific as you write your goals. (Remember: The "I'll of Putting Your Goals in Writing" is located in the specific ocean!) After you've written them and carried them around with you, and they're on the mirror in your bathroom, remember that if you stick to your initial desire, you can upgrade the goals for clarity or even rewrite them as often as you wish. Once you've created your written goals, you'll be able to go on to phase two of this all-important process in making your life all you want it to be.

This next important step is adding animation to your goals—giving them movement and life. I'm talking about vision. The more creative and positive your written goals, the more you assure a clear vision of accomplishment. Putting yourself into the vision—feeling, tasting, hearing, smelling, and knowing your success—is vitally important. Making yourself one with your vision and getting into it will help you envision your desired results. As ancient Proverbs in the Bible tell us, "As a man thinketh in his heart, so is he." Buddha said, "I am what I think, and I have become what I have thought." In modern language, this can be translated into: "What we visualize, we actualize," or "What we think about, we bring about." You want to put yourself into the race, see your victory, and feel the sting of the string snapping across your chest as you cross the finish line to collect your medal and the laurel of golden oak leaves just before you're hoisted up onto the shoulders of the joyous crowd.

Some people have negative goals. Although they might not realize it, they're putting out a lot of negative energy, which results in undesirable outcomes.

They can see things going wrong, and they step into that vision. These people can often be heard saying "I knew this would happen" as they refer to a disappointment. Visualization can be applied in either a positive or a negative direction. Therefore, results for one person might snowball into riches and fulfillment, another person might plummet into despair, and still another person might be more muddled today than yesterday.

This illustrates what we learned in Chapter 4 about how very creative you are. Let's say a young woman wants to grow up to be a sophisticated adult in the entertainment media. She might begin to visualize herself on television and start to act as if her goal is already actualized. As she takes on the behavior of the role models she sees, she can start manifesting results. Encouragement from others observing this behavior might further her on her way to achieving her goal. She might watch a lot of television and practice mimicking the people she sees on the screen. While she's developing a style of her own, she might take classes, play with the camera on her computer, and learn about makeup and what is most flattering to wear. By putting her goal in writing and having it in front of her all the time, she won't forget what she wants, even though life will come along with its many interruptions and distractions.

Playfully visualizing is creative and adds energy to your written goal. Visualization and energy produce powerful results, and can replace the agony of how difficult life seems to be. This will eliminate fruitless daydreaming and stimulate you to further your cause and take action.

The next step in this process is to create a schedule for what you need to do. At this point congratulate yourself, because you've already done what it takes to accomplish great things. You have motivation, written goals, and vision. Now simply move to the practical and ask yourself: "What logical steps must I take to accomplish my goal and realize my vision?" One of the best ways to develop your plan is to learn from others. Chances are that someone else has already had a similar goal and has been successful in achieving it. There is great value in studying the success of others.

As an example, let's imagine that your vision is to own a lucrative small business. Be specific that you want to own a dry-cleaning establishment. You would study the cleaning business and interview people who had successful cleaning businesses. You could go to work for a cleaning business and learn every phase of the operation. You might also take college classes on the finance and bookkeeping aspects of operating a small business. Soon, you'd have enough information to devise a practical plan to make your vision a reality.

To further clarify, imagine that you want to be a successful public speaker. Again, study success. Read about the lives of people such as Ronald Reagan, John Kennedy, and Abraham Lincoln, who were inspirational and influential through their speaking ability. Become involved in groups that train and support speakers, such as Toastmasters International. Finally, accept any invitation to speak to any group, large or small, to fine-tune your abilities.

With the goal and vision in mind, you need only study the practical steps that others who've been successful in whatever it is you want to accomplish have taken. This doesn't mean that you can't go beyond and surpass the accomplishments of those who've gone before you. Simply let others pave the way. Then, once you know all there is to know about your field of endeavor, new and creative avenues will open to you.

Once you've identified the practical steps to get what you want, you can begin to establish a time frame. The entrepreneurial-minded individual who wants to establish a dry-cleaning business might be looking at a five-year plan. The person will most likely spend several years working for someone else and taking classes. Further time would be spent selecting a location and establishing financing for the business. Our person who wants to be a speaker, on the other hand, might be looking at a shorter time frame. That person might set a goal of making the first presentation to a class or organization in weeks or months, with more elaborate presentations to be made later. Whatever the goal and vision, as you delineate the steps, set a time schedule. This will help you to be realistic, and to avoid discouragement and procrastination.

There is one important truth, however, about this step: There are no shortcuts. You can never get something without giving a fair equivalent. True success in any endeavor requires study and self-development to be all you can be. This is true whether you want to have a successful marriage, to be a loving parent, to achieve health, or to acquire money. The steps take work. They do, however, unfold in logical sequence when the vision is firmly in mind and in writing.

A good starting place to stimulate your creative ability is to ask yourself these questions:

> What do I want my love relationships to be?
> How do I want my body to manifest health?
> What do I want to look like one year from now?
> How much money do I want, and what kind of service would I like to provide in order to get it?

These are the four most important questions you might ever answer. The answers will set the process of becoming your own genie in motion. Decide what you want. Don't rely on fate and luck to determine your destiny. Your life can manifest qualities that give you a sense of integrity and that will inspire others. Think about what you want, know you have the power to create it, and then decide what you want. Then, read on. The remainder of this book will help you shape your thinking and gain the wisdom to actualize your results.

A Case History in "Calling": Arthur's Story

The first time I was aware of the power of goals, I was 19 years old and serving in the United States Navy. After surviving boot camp, I became a medical corpsman. I must have shown above-average stamina because, upon graduation, I was assigned to work on the locked psychiatric ward at the largest naval hospital in the world, in San Diego, California. I worked in that position until my four-year term of service was over, and I had many experiences that helped me to develop and mature.

The most unpleasant part of the job was night duty. We all had to do it, and this boring and cumbersome assignment came around about every four months. Our duties required that we muster at 9 p.m. for inspection, go do dinner in the dining hall, and report to work at 11 p.m. We got off work at 7 a.m., went to breakfast, mustered for another inspection, and were assigned to clean the bathrooms in the enlisted men's barracks. Our term of service was three weeks without a day off. The hardest part was staying awake all night and trying to get sleep during the day.

Today, I'm grateful for all the time I had without any distractions. I had just discovered the process of establishing goals and putting them in writing. I used my long hours in the dark to map out a plan for my future. I had to begin by deciding what I wanted, and, before I could put this in writing, I had to take responsibility for my thinking, which stimulated my creativity. Before I knew it, my catalog of possibilities was right in front of me. Knowing that I was a "spotlight person," I wanted to be in the atmosphere of performance. Having been in shows in school, I knew that I really enjoyed being in front of people. My original goal was to be in some form of show business.

After I put my goals in writing, I could see that it wasn't exactly what I wanted. I became aware that, although I wanted to be presenting to people, what I presented had to go deeper than a song or a joke. It was after I wrote my first goal that I realized I didn't want to be a performer; I wanted to be an inspirational presenter, something like the many ministers who had inspired and helped me all through my life.

At that point I felt unworthy of such an occupation. I knew I'd have to do a lot of research to see if I could achieve this goal. I spoke to my minister and asked him about having a calling. I thought this was like the heavens opening up, a beam of bright light falling on my head and shoulders, and the booming voice of

God saying: "Arthur, I have chosen you to become an ordained minister. Now go and do this thing I have called ye to do." My minister told me he had never received such a calling, but he soul searched and prayed about his decision, and when he knew it was right he pursued his dream. He suggested that I do the same. So I prayed and soul searched, and asked for a sign so that I would know without a doubt I could become what I so earnestly wanted to be.

The next Sunday, after attending worship services and volunteering as an usher at the church I attended, my path crossed that of the Reverend Marie Fleming, a retired Unity minister who served as the assistant to the senior minister. Her demeanor was stately and elegant, she dressed beautifully, and, when she prayed before the congregation on Sunday mornings, I had the feeling of being in the presence of someone very special. I deeply admired her, and when she said, "I've been watching you serve our church, and I think you would make a fine Unity minister," sure enough the heavens parted, the birds sang, and I was deeply touched. I had received my sign.

That night at the hospital, while working on the ward, I took a new, clean, white sheet of paper and started to change my life and have what I wanted. Exactly how I would make it happen wasn't as important at that point. Just knowing what I wanted was the most important building block to put in place. Because I had received my sign, I was certain that all the rest would follow just as miraculously.

I vividly remember mapping the order of the events that needed to occur before I would be ordained. I'd have to finish my tour of service to my country, which would take another three years and four months. During that time, I could get experience serving in my church. I could take correspondence courses with the parent organization through the Unity Correspondence School. There would be college and summer sessions at Unity Village near Kansas City, Missouri. I made a time line—a list of years and what needed to be accomplished in each year. Looking at my list, I felt as though it would take forever to reach my goal, but I knew I could and would do it.

By the time I finished my list, dawn's light was starting to stream through the bars of the windows of my world, but I knew I was no longer imprisoned by what could not be. I had taken responsibility, I knew what I wanted, I had a clearly defined goal, my goal was in writing, I could see myself experiencing the finished product, and I was willing to do the work. I am thankful for all the ingredients that helped me accomplish the groundwork that led to this epiphany and the development of my career. I trust that as you read about my success, you'll be inspired to use the ingredients I used to create your own success.

I am also reminded of another story about how thinking and beliefs affected my life in a different way.

A couple of friends of mine invited me to go on a ski trip with them to Mammoth Lakes, California. My first thought was: "I don't know how to ski, but I'm sure I'd enjoy it." So I signed up, paid my money, rented some skis, boots, and poles, packed up sweaters, hats, and gloves, and even purchased a pair of ski pants. I was all set to go!

Just as my friends said, the chartered bus trip was a party on wheels, our condo was warm and comfortable, and the mountain was beautiful. I signed up for my ski class and met with my fellow students at 9 a.m. Hans, our instructor, was a handsome, blond Norwegian. Among the people in the class were a family of four and two married couples; the rest of us were single, including me at the time. A lovely young woman named Julie and I seemed to hit it off.

As the lesson got under way, I fast discovered that it was terrifying to be sliding down a slippery, snow-covered hill with a bottomless edge looming up and not being able to stop. So, Hans's first instruction was how to stop ourselves by making "the wedge," a sort of duck-toed stance one forms with skis that creates additional friction, which helps beginning skiers maintain control until they feel comfortable skiing with the skis turned straight.

Hans had us make two columns facing each other, with a wide space between us. He had each of us sidestepping up the hill to get to the head of the line; there, we would form the wedge and ski down through the columns of students on each side. When we reached the bottom, we'd start sidestepping our way up back up to the starting position, form the wedge again, and then slide down the hill again until we reached the bottom.

We all did this until we all could stop successfully. For me, the experience was filled with flashbacks from my childhood—uneasy memories of learning something new, not feeling confident, and not being successful at first. I didn't like this feeling. What made it worse was that every time I got into the starting position, with the bottomless edge in full sight, Hans was looking at me. I was so nervous that I had to fight for the courage to put the tips of my skis together to make that wedge, and then push off and slide down the hill though the watching students while trying not to fall down. To make things even more difficult for me, every time I succeeded in my attempt, Hans didn't see me because he was talking to Julie. When I did a poor job of making the wedge and sliding down the hill, he noticed and commented about how I needed to stand up straighter, stop looking at my skis, pay attention, or whatever other criticism he could offer. In other words, when I did it right I didn't get credit, but when I wasn't perfect I got criticism.

Hans showed us how to get on the chairlift, which was just as terror-inducing and flashback-inducing for me as the sidestep-and-wedge lesson had been. By the time we broke for lunch, I wasn't just exhausted; I was carrying an overwhelming feeling of defeat. The cafeteria was filled with skiers who were obviously happy with themselves and the sport of skiing, but all I could hear were echoes from my past. I could hear teachers and coaches telling me all the things I was doing wrong, and I remembered how none of them ever seemed to see me or give me credit when I got it right.

At that point, I realized that I was in trouble. I couldn't go home because the bus wasn't leaving for three more days. I had paid all this money and rented all this equipment, and I was too frugal to waste the time and money. But, most of all, what would everyone from the bus and back at the condo think of my cowardice? I realized that I had to develop an interest in continuing my lessons (which would resume after lunch), and I had to muster up the belief that I could learn to ski.

I hurriedly finished my lunch, grabbed my skis and poles, got on the chairlift, and made the best wedges that anyone had ever made on Jill's Run at Mammoth Mountain. This isn't saying that the rest of the day was easy; the other lessons were at least as hard as the first ones, and by 3 p.m. I was exhausted. In addition, the pattern of Hans's not seeing when I got it right continued. But with every trip down the slope, I tried harder.

At the end of the day's final class, Hans called us all together and suggested that tomorrow we should take an "A" class. Then, he turned to Julie and me and said, "Arthur and Julie, I think tomorrow you should take a 'B' class." I felt depressed and angry. The anger turned to fury that for all my effort, all I got was a B, and everyone else got an A.

On the bus ride back to the condo and hot tub and during dinner, my fellow adventurers were all happy, and because they knew I had signed up for a full-day class that day, they enthusiastically said, "Oh, Arthur, don't you just love the skiing? How did you do in your class?" I honestly felt like saying I wished I was someplace else or that I hated skiing and I didn't think I'd ever be able to do it. But I couldn't bring myself to not speak the truth, so I said, "My teacher, Hans, suggested that tomorrow I take the B class."

The ribbing and rebuffs had I expected didn't happen. In

fact, I was astonished when they all started talking at once, saying things like this: "Wow! That's great! And after you finish your B class, you can take a C class, and then you can take a D class!"

The light dawned in my head, and I said, "You mean it goes the other way?" And they all said, "Yes. Didn't you know that?" And I said, "Not until just now."

Then I said, "You know, I love this skiing stuff, and I can't wait to get on the mountain tomorrow." The feeling was genuine once I became aware that my endeavors that day had resulted in success, not the failure I was basing on the echoes of my past. Best of all was realizing that the hard work and effort I had applied to accomplish my goal had not gone unrecognized.

Many wonderful opportunities in my life came from learning how to ski. The most important was when I met my wife, Virginia, who also loved to ski, and she invited me to go skiing with her. It was during that ski trip that we fell in love, and within a few months we were married. Other results from taking that first ski class were measured in fitness, feelings of success, a second-home ski cabin in Mammoth Lakes, California, teaching my two sons how to ski, and the ability to ski safely and with confidence. My adventures have taken me to many ski resorts in the United States as well as Italy, Switzerland, and France. Somehow I knew all these possibilities existed that first moment my friends invited me to hop on the tour bus, go to the mountain, and take a lesson.

Once you develop the skills of finding the interest and believing in the possibilities of the things you envision for you, you're ready to go to the next step: taking the time to decide what you want and deciding that you'll have it. You'll find the tools for this in our next chapter.

Your Map to "I'll Create My Goals and Put Them in Writing"

Put your goals in writing, and develop the capacity to visualize your results.

Add animation to your goals, giving them movement and life.

Create a schedule for what you need to do.

Know the practical steps you'll need to take to get to your desired results.

Be prepared to do the work and enjoy the results.

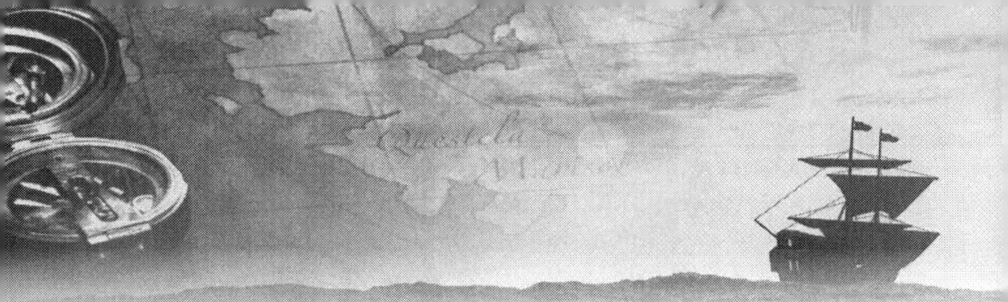

Chapter 8

Go Fast, Like a Tortoise

Slow but sure moves the might of the gods.
~ Euripides (ca. 480–406 BCE),
Greek writer of tragedies

THE winner's circle is full of tortoises. This elite group of victors crossed the finish line way ahead of the overconfident hares. Aesop wrote about this. A lesser-known tortoise victory was relayed in Zeno's Paradoxes, one of which is "The Paradox of Achilles and the Tortoise." In this paradox, Achilles is in a footrace with the tortoise, and he allows the tortoise a head start of 100 meters. Whenever Achilles reaches a spot where the tortoise has been, he still has farther to go; he can never overtake the tortoise. The tortoise is always ahead of Achilles, and he can also outrun the hare. Again, the tortoise wins.

Looking at what the hare teaches us, we learn not to be overconfident, or to brag, or to get distracted, or to go off course. (Actually, I think one of the reasons the hare lost the race is because he got distracted and fooled around with the Energizer Bunny.) The illustration of the tortoise teaches the values of taking your time, moving forward at a steady pace, not being distracted, and keeping your goal in mind at all times.

In elementary school, I remember my teacher placing a bean

in a glass jar between the glass and a wet paper towel. Each day the class would add water to the bottom of the jar, which would be absorbed by the paper towel. This moist environment accommodated the sprouting bean, whose roots started to become visible and whose first little leaf started to sprout at its top. Before long we were planting the sprouted beans in soil. I learned the importance of being patient and how much time some things take to reach completion.

Identifying with the tortoise and discovering the importance of moving slowly might cause us to experience a reaction that says: "But I must accomplish this quickly. I can't go slowly. I want to see results." This might be a good time to look at our choices and rearrange our reactions. When you take charge of your reactions, it's like you're planting seeds. You control your reaction, which you could think of as a seed. We need to understand that once something happens to us, we have control over our reactions to it. We create our world through how we deal with our reactions. Each reaction or thought acts like a seed to grow that thought or reaction, and it snowballs to become better or worse. You can look back and trace how a thought became a reality, or you can focus on where you are and how to get where you want to be.

You don't pull into a gas station and ask the attendant, "How did I get here?" You ask for directions to where you're going. It's important that you know you can proceed from where you are. You can create a new tomorrow with your brightest thoughts and interests of today. This creative process needs to be enjoyed and thought of as a journey from where you are to where you want to be.

Wherever you go, go with all your heart.

~ Confucius (551–479 BCE), philosopher

You can make your progress from here to your completed goal a wondrous experience and enjoy each step along the way. Taking charge of your reaction to be in too much of a hurry will remove a lot of pressure and give you time to grow into what you want to become. It's important to know this when you write your goals and make a time line for their completion.

A Case History in Slowly Reaching Your Goals: David and Marjorie's Story

David and Marjorie were a young, married couple living in war-torn London. They never knew what the next day would bring, and there were blackouts, air raids, and nightly bombings. David served in the Royal Air Force and had to be away from home for weeks at a time. Marjorie and many other young British women worked at an underground bomb-making factory, assembling explosives that would be dropped on the enemy. The work they did was tedious, and the smallest mistake could cost many lives. Walking through the bombed-out rubble of London on her way to work gave Marjorie a vivid picture of how the explosives she was helping produce would create the same damage for those who had damaged London.

David and Marjorie had little time to spend together, but when they were together they made the most of every minute. They especially liked taking walks and dancing, and when they had a little extra money they went to the local pub, which overflowed with servicemen and civilians. They joined in the singing and fun while everyone tried to make the most of every moment in a world where no one was certain how many moments the future held. Often these happy times were shattered by the blast of a bomb and the screaming of warning sirens, followed by people scurrying home in the dark to safety.

The thing David and Marjorie did best together was dream

of a time ahead filled with peace and tranquility. Whether they knew it or not, they were setting goals for their future. Their wish list included meaningful jobs in line with the level of British life they were born into. They envisioned themselves moving to the United States, away from England and the scars of war, with enough money to be comfortable.

They understood that it would take time to reach their goals, yet they saw that long span of time as a kind of necessary incubation period. Talking about these goals every time they were together helped them escape the brutal reality of war. Even so, reaching their goals seemed impossible—or, if it were possible, it would take forever. There didn't seem to be anything they could do to make these goals real; they could only dream, so dream they did. They were moving, slowly, toward reaching their goals, whether they knew it or not.

One evening, just days after the war was over, David and Marjorie were on their familiar route. Suddenly, all the lights, long-darkened by the blackout restriction, came on. For the first time in years, Parliament and Big Ben were flooded with light. Not only was there light, but the bells of Big Ben began loudly clanging out the hour.

Of all the places to be in London when the lights came on, they were there. David and Marjorie believed this was the start of their dreams coming true. They took this magical moment as a sign that all would be well. Then and there, they decided to accelerate their efforts to create what they desired.

They found their way to America and settled in the Chicago area. A couple of cold and snowy winters later, they moved to warm and sunny California. They found Los Angeles too crowded, so they moved to the San Diego area, into a small apartment in La Mesa. They were willing to work at just about anything, and they found odd jobs to bring in enough money to pay the bills and cover the rent. They realized that as soon as they started to speak, their British accents impressed Americans.

Their new friends treated them like royalty, and they were warmly received wherever they went. They took long walks in their new warm and sunny home, and they were happy.

Knowing they'd have future needs that their present income wouldn't provide, they continued the practice of setting goals, talking about what they wanted, and dreaming of the possibilities of a better life. They were patient with the process of dreams coming true, and did all they could to put a little money aside. They were moving slowly toward their goal, but they were moving.

They furnished their small apartment with furniture they found at yard sales and through newspaper ads, repairing and refinishing the discarded belongings of others, and making them attractive and desirable. David did the refinishing, and Marjorie sewed and reupholstered. With the encouragement of friends and neighbors, they rented a small store and continued refurbishing used furniture to sell. Business was slow, and they weren't doing all that well, but they held onto their dream.

One day, after a particularly slow week in the shop, David and Marjorie were feeling low. Spending money they didn't have wasn't a good idea, but they needed cheering up. They put on their best clothes and drove to downtown San Diego to splurge by enjoying high tea at the palatial US Grant Hotel. They fit right in with the crowd of tea-sipper types who enjoyed the traditional Thursday high tea in the hotel's beautiful Palm Room. As usual, they were cordial to the people around them. They noticed a couple of elderly women who looked like something out of a novel, dressed in classic clothing, complete with hats and gloves, who looked refined although outdated. David and Marjorie spoke to them, and again the British accent did its magic. The four had a charming conversation, and David and Marjorie felt at home enjoying tea and crumpets and chatting with others who seemed part of a world they had known a long time ago. They went home promising to return some Thursday in the near future.

Weeks went by before they realized it was teatime again. The Grant Hotel and its elegant Palm Room were as beautiful as always, the teacarts were overflowing with goodies, and the elegant crowd gathered, and they were delighted to see the two elderly women. While they visited, the women announced that they had to leave, because it would take them a while to walk from the hotel to the ferry, which they would ride across the San Diego Bay and then have a short walk to their home in Coronado.

David and Marjorie were amazed that these two women would be on foot. They seemed too unsteady and overdressed to accomplish such a feat. They urged the women to stay longer and enjoy the tea and snacks, and said that they would gladly drive them home. The women accepted their offer, and as the conversation continued, David and Marjorie told the women their life story. The women were impressed with David and Marjorie's adventurous journey to the United States, and at some point, they said their names were May and Jayne. May was the older sister, and she was in charge of Jayne. They had lived in Coronado for many years after moving to California from New York City. After their husbands' deaths they shared a house. When it was time to go, all four of them got into the car and drove to the ferry, which took them across the bay to Coronado. As they reached the house, David and Marjorie were astonished that it was so large and elegant, even though there were signs of neglect. May and Jayne said that they would like to welcome them inside through the front door, but they couldn't get it open, so they would all have to go through the kitchen entrance.

Inside, David and Marjorie commented on how cold the house was. The women said it had been cold for weeks, and they thought the heating system must be broken. David asked to be taken to the front door to see if he could help open it. Once there he immediately identified the problem. So much mail had been delivered through the letter slot in the door that the door was blocked. He explained this to the women, and they said their vision was so poor and the house so dark that they hadn't noticed the mail piling up. They asked David to pick up the avalanche, and as he did he noticed warning envelopes from utility companies and what looked like important letters with Wall Street return addresses. He brought these to the women, who again said that their lack of vision and lighting had impaired their ability to open and read the mail.

At that moment, David and Marjorie realized that the house was dark and cold because the electricity had been turned off. They politely asked if the ladies had the funds to pay the bills, and both May and Jayne laughed. May said, "Oh, we have plenty of money in the bank. We just can't find our checkbook." The couple realized that it wasn't safe for the ladies to live in these circumstances, and they offered to come back the next day and help them to get the electricity turned back on, make bank deposits, and pay the big stack of bills. The thankful women agreed.

What seemed a day's work turned into a week and then a second week. David and Marjorie were just volunteering, with no expectation of being compensated for their time. While David answered the mail, Marjorie helped clean and organize. All four got in the car and made numerous trips to the bank to make large deposits. The women were so appreciative of David and Marjorie's help that they offered them the job of taking care of their household and of them. Before long Jayne and May had been to their doctor for the first time in years, were taking medications that were a boost to their health, and had new glasses. For the first time in years, they could see, they had regular meals thanks to Marjorie's cooking, they were living in a house that had light and heat, and they were very happy.

David and Marjorie were happy, too. The dreams they had of quality and meaningful employment with perks had been realized. They enjoyed restoring the women to the lifestyle they had enjoyed before their decline. They went to the opera (one of the sisters' favorite things to do) and to black-tie events, one of which May had started when she first came to Coronado. The four of them traveled to visit the site of the women's family home in New York City and then to visit David and Marjorie's roots in London en route to a sunny fortnight in the French Riviera. Eventually the women had the court appoint David and Marjorie as their official guardians, which had all four of them set for life. And almost every Thursday, the four of them enjoyed high tea in the Palm Room at the Grant Hotel.

David and Marjorie didn't reach the goals they set for themselves quickly. Although the pace seemed tortoise-slow, they did reach what they had aimed for and more. Their story reminds us to set our goals, go over them time and again, fix them firmly in our minds, vividly visualize ourselves in them, do the work required, and move at a tortoise pace, enjoying each phase of the process as we move closer to our goals.

Your Map to "I'll Go Fast Like a Tortoise"

Have your goals in writing.

Give yourself plenty of time to accomplish the work that needs to be done.

Know that to have quality results, you'll have to invest quality time and that the process is like planting seeds and should be enjoyed.

Watch your efforts grow like seeds.

Enjoy feeling the changes and the increase of the good that you experience.

Keep moving slowly but surely toward your goal.

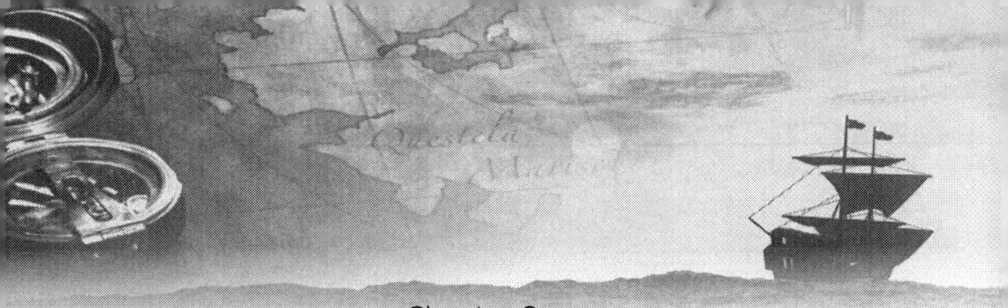

Chapter 9

Become Magnetic: Become What You Want, and Attract Help

You are a living magnet. What you attract into your life is in harmony with your dominant thoughts.

~ Brian Tracy (b. 1944),
motivational speaker and author

IN this chapter we'll explore the magic that happens when you combine thought and creativity. That magic is called the Law of Magnetism. And it is the next phase that automatically responds to the activity of creative thought.

On my 59th birthday, I had an epiphany about how I wanted to look and how I wanted my life to be arranged when I turned 60 in a year. This was not a shallow experience, because I spent considerable time and energy thinking about my goals and commitment, and realizing and believing I could create all that I desired. It was at this time that my catalog of possibilities arrived. This wasn't a literal catalog but a mind full of possibilities in picture form. As I leafed through it, I could clearly see what choices were possible.

Immediately, the Law of Magnetism started to work for me. I remembered advice I had received during my 59 years of life. I was fortunate to attract information about how to reach my goals. The best way to describe it is to say that it felt like magic. An important thing about this magical law is that, if one doesn't activate it, the catalog never arrives. This might explain why some individuals seem to have results and gather life's rewards, while others who might seem more capable do not.

I was quite familiar with the Law of Attraction and had received many catalogs in the past. Although I knew about the Law of Attraction, I was about to have many wonderful things occur for my benefit via the Law of Magnetism. This is the law that sends the ideas and direction to you that you need just when you need them. Honoring their receipt is important, because the source of inspiration responds to your response. If there is no response and follow-through from you to the inspiration the law sends, your subscription is immediately put on hold. When there is response, more and more inspiration comes. The receipt of my latest catalog at that time seemed more important than at any time in the past.

The images that appeared in my epiphany were of me attending my 60th birthday party. The party would be a gift to me from my wife, Virginia, and it promised to be a splendid affair with catered food, a live band, dancing, and dining, all in the comfort of my home. I was expecting about 75 guests (which translates into about 35 gifts). The images I had included me looking trim, slim, and handsomely dressed, having a wonderful time, and hearing my guests tell me: "You don't look like you're 60 years old." The epiphany also seemed to say: "While you're at it, let's take this creativity thing a step further, and why not make an accomplishment in some unknown area so you can anticipate hearing people say 'I understand that during the past year you've made quite an accomplishment in _____ (the unknown area of _____).'"

At that point, I drew a blank. Accomplishment in what? But the assurance came that the blank would be filled in as and if I continued. Everything within me agreed with the images and possibilities. All I had to do was commit to doing my part, so I did. And as soon as I did, the Law of Attraction went to work for me.

At the moment of my epiphany I was in the gym in my home, doing my regular workout. As the law kicked in, I realized that to make my dream of celebrating my success at the party come true, I needed to pump it up in my workout. I could distinctly hear the advice of several past personal trainers: "You have the muscle and the build to look like these pictures you show us of how you want to look. All you have to do is bite the bullet and do the work." Recalling that advice, weights in hand, I committed to doing the work while realizing that, if I overdid it, I would cause muscle pain that would take days to repair and that would sabotage my efforts. So I increased my weights just enough to get the workout I needed without hurting myself and disrupting the progress I was committed to making.

The frequency of inspirational moments magnetically became a big part of my makeover formula that fell into my plan. One memorable incident occurred while I was visiting Carol, the lovely woman who cleans my teeth three times a year. Because we spend so much time together I consider her a friend. I really enjoy our one-way conversations, during which I'm limited to a few grunts and some abbreviated "uh-huhs." On this occasion, while Carol was working away, she said she was training for an upcoming half-marathon race. With great enthusiasm, she spoke of the several thousand other people who'd be running with her, the exhilaration of an early-morning start, the accomplishment of crossing the finish line, and the celebration at the beer garden.

As soon as I had an opportunity to rinse, I asked, "How did you find out about this race? I've never heard of it before." She told me about a magazine published every few months that lists all the races in the San Diego area. "Go just down the street to this running store, Movin Shoes, and pick up a copy," Carol suggested. "Then look through it, and pick out the race you want to do, and sign up."

I mentioned that I'd been running for years, but I wasn't sure I could run 13.11 miles. She assured me that I could run at my own pace, that there was no reason to be anxious, that it was fun, and that people who were older than I was and in worse shape often ran with little difficulty.

I left the dentist's office, and while my hand was on the door handle of my car, I was thinking, "I'd like to have a copy of that *Race Place Magazine*. One of these days, I'll go to that store and pick up a copy."

Then, honoring the source of the epiphany, I said to myself, "No, not someday, but now, because I'm really serious about reaching my goal of transforming my appearance, energy level, and accomplishment by my 60th birthday party."

So I went directly to the running store, and as I stepped inside, it was like Alice falling through the looking glass. I left the store with the magazine, new Mizuno running shoes, and a new interest and skill to develop that would supercharge my goals and add to the quality of my life in ways I had never dreamed possible. On that fateful day, my thoughts and creativity, stimulated by the Law of Attraction, helped me to attract my own catalog of possibilities. From my catalog I could choose what I wanted.

Your catalog has probably already arrived and given you several nudges, in fact. One way you know it's arrived is that you start seeing a result you'd like to create all around you. If it's fitness you want to increase, perhaps you see more fit people everywhere you go. Or perhaps gym advertisements are more obvious, and the flyers you get in the mail are more noticeable. This positive urge is saying to you, "Here is a possibility for you to claim. Are you willing to do the work, and do you really want the results you've been dreaming of?"

Now, I'd like to tell you the rest of the story, and highlight the 10 steps I discovered during my process of reaching my goals and creating the results I longed for.

The story begins on the fourth day of October 2002, my 59th birthday. Beginning a new trip around the sun has always been a special day for me. On my birthday, I always awaken with gratitude for a completed year, and I feel energized about the possibilities my new year can bring. This is a habit I've had all my life. So on this birthday I awakened early, like I always do, and after a cup of coffee I went to the gym in my home and started my regular, 30-minute morning weightlifting workout. Later I would go running with Virginia.

My head was full of thoughts about the year ending and the year ahead. I realized that this would be the last year of my fifth decade. I thought back about the past year and wondered what I could create in this year that would carry me into and through my sixth decade. I had a sense of now or never to begin doing the things that needed to be done to have the quality of life I longed for.

In my sixth decade, I would retire from the ministry I had founded some 36 years earlier, and my thoughts went to what I'd be doing in retirement and what my future accomplishments would be. My thoughts also covered a wide spectrum that involved the questions of "How do I want to wind up my career in ministry?" and "What's the legacy I'd like to leave behind?" I had a desire to move forward and go out with a bang at the same time. While I went through my weightlifting exercises, I thought, "This can be a year of transformation for me."

As these thoughts flooded my awareness, an inspiration started to hatch within me. This sense of possibility started to grow, and I began thinking: "This is my last year in this decade, and it's important to me to create happy endings. The way something ends carries over and flavors the way the new beginning starts."

So I asked myself, "Why not make this the best year of your life—a transformational year of your life?" Then I asked, "What would the life you'd like to be living look like? How would you get from here to there? How much will it take in the costs of energy and time? Do you have the time, and do you really have the interest and desire?"

As my workout continued, I noticed that my thoughts were jumping around. Knowing I had hit on something very close and personal to my desires, my thoughts leapt to my wife's plans for that evening. I knew that Virginia was going to take me out to dinner, which would be a quiet celebration, because she had planned a party for my 60th birthday.

More questions came: "At my party, what do I want to look like one year from today? What do I want the guests to see in me that they're not seeing now? What claim to fame would I like to have that I don't have today? And what recognition can I expect?"

A flood of answers poured into my awareness, and what I like to call my Higher Self began to speak. This still, small voice asked me some important questions: "Do you really want to make this the best year of your life? What if you really did the work that needs to be done on your consciousness, on your thinking, on your habits, on your discipline, and on your body and health? What if you made this your year of transformation? What if you attended your 60th birthday party and radiated a state of consciousness and awareness, and looked really fit and good? What if your guests said, 'We hear you've taken up something new and exciting, and you're making great strides forward and expanding your sphere of accomplishments. Congratulations.'?"

Then I asked back, "Where do I begin?"

The pattern I had been living and teaching for the previous

59 years emerged to help the epiphany, that sudden moment of insight, break through.

As I was exiting my fifth decade and entering my sixth, I would make this a transformational year. My belief in the possibility was strong, and this was when my thinking launched me into orbit. I didn't know how I was going to do it, but I knew I was going to do it. I could see the result I desired, and although the vision wasn't crystal clear, the potential and the feeling I wanted to create were on fire inside me. For the rest of my workout, through my run, and for the remainder of the day, my thoughts were consumed by the possibilities before me.

With the epiphany came the acceptance that I had a lot of work to do. I needed to use this power to reorganize my thinking about how to make this my transformational year. I'd have to evaluate my thoughts, discover what might be holding me back, and determine which thoughts I could use to propel me forward. I had a lot of thinking and rethinking to do.

As a creative person, I found that this stimulus caused by my epiphany started my creative juices flowing, and I was energized to create a new workout routine. Immediately the Law of Attraction delivered my catalog of possibilities and inspiration. I could vividly see myself at my 60th birthday party. I could vividly hear and see the response to my year of transformation from my friends and guests. I knew the next step would be revealed to me, but I had to keep moving.

What I had to confront at that point were the big questions: Was I really interested, or was this just a passing fancy, *and* did I really believe I could accomplish this goal? For several days I struggled to find the interest and the belief. I had been working out and lifting weights for years, I had had several personal trainers, and I was interested in building muscle and creating a handsome body. But my interest was shallow. I did the work and I lifted the weights, but I never gained the results I desired due to a lack of genuine interest. To have the results I really desired, I would have to deepen my interest.

At that point, I again remembered the personal trainer's words: "You have the build, height, and muscle to look like those pictures you showed me in the magazine of the guy you'd like to look like. All you have to do to have that look is bite the bullet and do the work." Then I remembered asking him: "What does 'bite the bullet' look like to you?" And he said, "That's when you just buckle down and do the work. If you really went for it and lifted the weight and did the aerobic exercises and managed your diet, you'd have that look you want in a few months."

I had heard these words before, but I hadn't seriously heeded them until then. The power of my thinking and my creativity attracted my catalog. Each of these elements became the driving force of my epiphany, and the opportunity to make this my year of transformation pulled me into a "bite the bullet" state of mind. I found more earnest determination than I had ever known before. As I was sensitive to this determination, I realized I had been exposed to people who were so determined that they lost sight of the fun and adventure they could be having if they hadn't been so determined. With this example in mind and knowing that I had one year to reach my goal, I decided to curb my determination and enthusiasm with patience and a steady work ethic, and apply myself to slow but sure persistence, each and every day, for the next year.

This brought me to a place where I decided to set this goal and work toward it until I accomplished it. I would have what I wanted, I would build what I wanted, and I knew that I could create what I wanted. I was deeply and genuinely interested, and I believed that I could reach this goal.

Reaching this conclusion and growing through this process took about 10 to 14 days. During these days I had many things to do, but I took the time to think this through. As I did my thinking I had to confront limiting thoughts and fuel my ambition with possibility thoughts. There was a flood of activity that I had to organize in my brain while life went on all around me.

From the first day, I had my goals in writing. Knowing the importance of seeing them morning and night, I posted them on the mirror in my bathroom. I took the liberty of editing them every time I saw them to sharpen my focus and to clarify exactly how I wanted them to materialize. I kept a copy of my goals with me at all times in my shirt pocket over my heart. I found myself editing them and reading them several times during the day. I firmly believe this grounded me in my goals. As the writing of my goals became more specific, my vision of their being complete in my life became sharper.

Writing out my goals and holding the vision of them as completed had helped me serve more efficiently as the CEO of the church I had founded. My family life and my work life were exceedingly full. In my career I had counseling appointments, weekly religious instruction classes, Sunday lessons to prepare, and weddings, funerals, and functions to attend. At home I had my personal life with my family and friends, social obligations, and my workouts and running. All these activities kept me busy, and at times they seemed to offer an excuse for me to not stick to my goals. These activities often involved so much thinking and energy that at times it seemed as though I was too tired or distracted to keep my goals in mind. But the vision and the pressure on me to complete this process in one year was so alive in me that I kept on keeping on.

At that point I felt as though I was over the top. I was committed, I had a clear vision of what I wanted, my goals were in writing, and I was determined. Then I noticed the magical activity of the Law of Magnetism taking place in my life. I had segregated my goals into seven specific areas. Each area seemed to draw magical happenings that I would have never dreamed possible and that I had never been aware of before. Determination drew these results and this information to me, and if I hadn't been determined and had the vision, this information wouldn't have been available to me. I had been running for years, both by myself and with my wife. We enjoyed our running time together, but we didn't really run as much as we jogged. Speed and distance weren't as important as socializing. But as I gradually realized that running would help burn all my stored calories and fat, and that running could transform my appearance to appear more energetic and youthful and create the success I wanted to show at my birthday party, I began to apply myself and ran farther and faster. I didn't forget about the principle of going at a turtle's pace rather than the faster rabbit; I simply began to increase my distance and speed slowly, by a little bit each week. Eventually I was running farther and faster, and Virginia—noting my progress and my physical changes in appearance—started running farther and faster with me. We could still maintain our social interaction, but at the same time we could go farther and faster, burn more calories, and gain health.

The Law of Magnetism drew other sources of help to me. Each year at the time of my birthday I have my annual medical and dental examinations. During this time I had the chat with Carol, which led me to a copy of *Race Place Magazine* and that new pair of running shoes.

This isn't saying that the path to my outcome was easy, but for those 365 days I progressed steadily and slowly toward my goal. On my 60th birthday, I celebrated the beginning of a new decade having reached my goals. Just as in my vision, as I greeted my birthday guests, they sounded sincere as they said in various ways: "You don't look like you're 60 to me." "I understand you've become a runner and that you've done a bunch of half-marathons." "You've lost a lot of weight, and you look really fit, trim, energetic, and young." All of it was just as I had imagined. I had reached my goal, acquired a new level of esteem, and set a pace for my new year, for my retirement, and for my new decade.

In summary, this was my route into terra incognita:

As you'll recall, it began with an epiphany. On my 59th birthday I asked myself what I wanted my 60th birthday to look like. The answer came back as a clear vision of what I could create. At that point, I found I had the interest and I believed I could accomplish this goal. So, I decided to go for it.

I put my desired goal in writing. The areas of my goal were family and other relationships, health, prosperity, mind, career, creativity, and spirit.

I made the decision and commitment to do it and to take the time necessary each day to do all I could do that day to reach my goal.

I made appointments with myself and kept them. Committed to going at a turtle's pace, I started. I began to get results that went beyond my wildest dreams: I burned more than 35 pounds of stored fat, gained over 15 pounds of muscle, and started competing in and winning races. At my annual medical examination, when my cholesterol and other blood levels came back, I had tangible proof it had been the year of transformation I desired it to be. I attracted the support I needed. I saw measurable results in my work and career. I increased my prosperity, I increased my esteem, and I started getting help from unexpected sources. If I hadn't had the epiphany I would have been sad, suffered low self-esteem, and had more fat, and my unproductive habits would have increased. The most damaging of all the effects of having a dream and not adhering to it would have been being angry with myself. This would have made me difficult to be around, and I would probably have eaten comfort foods to cushion my feelings and become fatter. I would have taken my anger out on my family and others. All of these qualities would have made me feel bad and be unpleasant to be around.

I firmly believe you can go from fable to fabulous. The fable

I'm referring to is Aesop's fable about the tortoise and the hare. You remember that the hare hopped all over the place and was so confident he was faster than the tortoise that he wasted time and lost the race. Clearly he wasn't determined. He was also a bit narcissistic and superior in his thinking. He probably hadn't put his goals in writing and lacked a vivid vision of winning the race. Before the race, he probably didn't do the visualization work of feeling the sting of the string snapping across his chest as he hopped across the finish line.

But the tortoise did. The tortoise also had vision and perseverance, and was goal-oriented and blessed with a level of stick-to-itiveness that kept him on course as he slowly but surely made his way to the finish line to complete his goal. He took his time and made every step count. He didn't lose his focus, and he transformed his reputation with himself and others into that of a winner. Such results are known as fabulous. (Or is that *fable*-ous?)

As I mentioned in the story about my hygienist having turned me on to running races, the same kinds of events happened over and over during the year I gave myself to this project. From the start, I knew it would take time and that the results I desired wouldn't appear quickly. So I decided to move toward my goal at a turtle's pace. Because this was an important goal, and I had it in writing, I activated the Law of Attraction and the Law of Magnetism.

> *Today you are a magnet, for infinite abundance, divine intelligence, and unlimited love. Actually this has always been true.*
>
> ~ Mike Dooley (b. 1961), inspirational author

When you do your part and put all the ingredients for success in place—including written goals, determination, and plenty of time—you start a flow of magic that comes into your life to help you on your way.

For instance, shortly after my 59th birthday, Virginia took me on a six-day Mexican Riviera cruise. While on board the cruise ship, in addition to working out in the gym and running around the deck every day, I attended a lecture given by the cruise spa staff about skin care and weight loss. When I went to the seminar I had no idea I was about to learn something that would prove to be a big aid to my success: a toxic cleansing of the body. Naturally, they had a product on board for sale that was guaranteed to cleanse your body of all toxins and cause you to lose that fat tire around your middle. With the lecture came a free test to measure toxicity and body fat. I knew my current weight and how much I wanted to weigh on my 60th birthday, but until that point I was unaware of fat tests. I made an appointment to have the test done, which resulted in the knowledge of what percentage of my body was fat.

The spa staff person, Jake, gave me a brief course in body fat. He told me that athletes in their prime often have eight- to nine-percent body fat. And he told me that 18- to 20-percent body fat is normal and that I had a 26-percent body fat count.

Although I didn't like hearing this, I was grateful to have a starting point for reaching my goal. Within the first month of my 12-month journey, I had gained valuable information to make my efforts over the next 11 months more successful. Jake also told me that if I were earnest and disciplined about my running and my weightlifting exercises, I'd burn off a large percentage of my body fat. He also highly recommended the toxic cleansing program. After thinking about it for a couple of days and coming back to ask him several questions, I purchased the product, which consisted of pills to take over a three-month period. Within three months of taking the cleansing pills, running, and weightlifting, I went from 26-percent body fat to 16-percent body fat. During the remaining months I worked diligently and reduced the number to eight-percent body fat, so on my 60th birthday, as I made my "debut" at my party, I had reached the same percentage of body fat that athletes in their prime possess. The guests at my birthday party noticed this change in my appearance and responded with that phrase I wanted to hear: "You don't look 60 to me."

Again, it's important to point out that this process took time—an entire year. And it's important to emphasize that all the time it took was worth the results I created for myself, and that pleased me. This not only took time, but it also took money for the cleansing pills and several other nutrients and supplements that helped me realize my dream. Let me emphasize here it's not that taking a pill can help you reach your goals. It took a considerable amount of time and determination, putting the goals in writing, and then working as hard as I've ever worked on anything to create the results I wanted—results I've maintained for eight years.

Not only is it important to do the foundation work, but it's also important to look for ways to do what needs to be done. This often brings the opportunity to do things you've never done before. It would have been easy for me to lie in a lounge chair by the pool sipping a mai tai instead of going to the spa lecture. Because of my determination and the vivid images of what I wanted, and because my goals were in writing, and I read them morning and night and carried them with me in the pocket of my shirt even on vacation, I couldn't miss the spa lecture. Because I went, and because I had goals and a vision of my expectations already in place, I heard exactly what I needed to hear, which sparked me to do exactly what I needed to do, resulting in making headway I would have never dreamed of if I hadn't established my goals and had chosen to sit in a lounge chair that day.

It's important to do the foundation work, place yourself in line to make new discoveries, and be ready to pay the price. Be prepared to discover results that will keep you on track as they amaze you.

In this yearlong adventure, I maintained the same attitude of discovery I had had at the spa. I constantly discovered ideas and information that would apply to each area, and that inspired me to do the work necessary to eliminate old beliefs and create new ones. I had to eliminate old habits and create new ones in order to have a sense of success. Slowly but surely, I saw goals coming to fruition. Knowing how far I had come and how far I had to go with my time limit in full view helped me have hindsight and perspective that gave me a deep sense of progress without a sense of frustration. I knew I was getting things done that would benefit my vision, and I persevered. My successes nourished me with energy, vision, and stamina to keep doing all the things I knew were necessary to arrive at my destination.

My adventures included establishing physical habits as well as invisible habits like discipline, thinking more positively, and always being receptive to beneficial ideas and inspiration turned to "on." I also noticed there was work to be done in the area I like to call challenges. Quite often, I came up against a wall that I felt was holding me back from making the progress I was accustomed to making. I found that to get over, around, or through this wall, I had to do a lot of work on myself.

Information and advice come to one who is in motion. Our goals and our dreams are waiting for our thoughts and creativity to set us into motion toward them. Once we're in motion, the Law of Magnetism brings us advice and information to further us on our way. To anyone who's the couch-potato type, at first this probably won't make a lot of sense. But those who choose to move forward know exactly what I'm talking about. If you can see the result and commit to it, begin to take the steps to get to that result, all that you need will be added to you along the way. This is what made my journey so delightful, and to this day I'm thankful for the guidance, information, and support I gathered.

I collected knowledge in the areas of diet and exercise, and I was introduced to the world of serious running. Since that time I've been in over 40 half-marathons, and many more races and charity events. In addition, I learned about nutrition and diet, supplements, fat burners, and nutrients, all of which helped to change the shape of my body as well as my mind. This is what made my journey so delightful.

Your Map to "I'll Become Magnetic"

See yourself as a magnet. Develop the belief that you draw to you exactly what you need when you need it.

Always be on the lookout for inspiration that will nudge you toward your success.

Act on the inspiration you attract. Taking action will guarantee more guidance in the future.

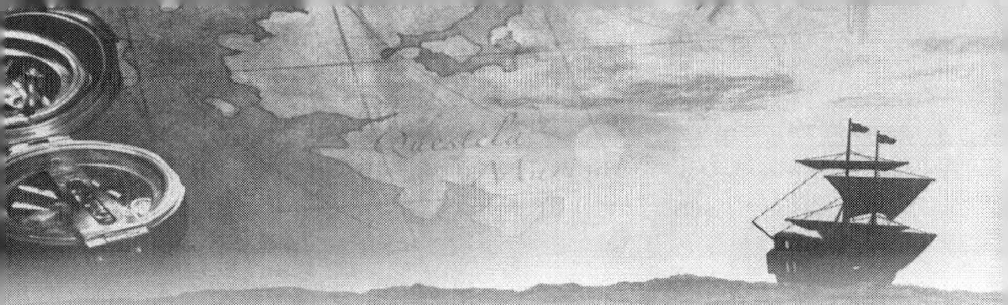

Chapter 10

Do the Work, Let Go of the Experience, and Keep the Lesson

Always do what you are afraid to do.
~ Ralph Waldo Emerson (1803–1882),
American essayist, lecturer, and poet

THIS chapter offers information to help you shape your thinking to benefit from the experiences you have encountered and the lessons you have learned. This step in your process of charting your way through terra incognita is where you really get your work done. It is very much like labor to manage your thoughts and stay on track. Let me share some ideas about the deeper work that has to be done on your life lessons.

When you take charge of your thinking and creativity and put your goals in writing, it's as though you're planting seeds. You've taken action, you've started to make things happen, and you've become sensitive to the control you have over those things. Your reactions are like seeds. We create our world through how we think about our world. Each reaction or thought acts like a seed to grow that thought or reaction, and the thought or reaction snowballs to become better or worse. It's inspiring to know that you can proceed from where you are to any place you want to be. It doesn't take magic; it takes hard work and determination. Working on your deeper issues will help you create a new tomorrow with your brightest thoughts and interests of today.

The same process applies to the major challenges in life. In an earlier chapter, I used as an example the goal of having a healthy love relationship. I suggested that, without condemning, blaming, or judging others, you take responsibility for the kind of relationships you created in the past. Then you take responsibility for creating the quality of relationships you want in the future.

Now that we understand the importance of taking our time, we can expect the Law of Magnetism to start working for us. As happened to me when I took that cruise, you attract information that you need—guidance you'll appreciate but that you never expected or knew anything about. Why? Because you've done so much work, you're ready for and have attracted the input you need to reach your goal.

Let's explore this idea that you can draw specific information, results, and events into your life with enough focus and concentration. Your thinking and enthusiasm for your goal create a kind of skeleton to which everything comes and sticks.

We know this is so, because we've learned that your thoughts are the most powerful thing you have going for you. With them, you create the world in which you want to live, work, and play. Knowing what you want makes you ready to put your vision into action.

You've set goals. You know what you want. You can visualize the result. You're motivated to take responsibility for your life. Problems and challenges should stop, right? Wrong! The universe simply isn't set up that way. Life will continue to offer a succession of challenges. It's helpful if you think of these challenges as lessons.

Let's explore life's lessons and discover how we can manage problems, setbacks, and challenges. To begin, I like this quote:

From error to error, one discovers the entire truth.
~ Sigmund Freud (1856–1939),
founder of psychoanalysis

The dictionary defines *lesson* as a reading or exercise assigned to a pupil to be studied. Life is full of lessons. A lesson presents something we need to learn in order to progress and evolve.

A lesson is presented to a student in a classroom. The student studies the material and its applications. Examples are offered. The student is then able to take the basic concept and apply it to a variety of new situations.

The same is true for each of us as our problems and challenges come up in life. We study the situation to understand the meaning. Once the reason for the problem is revealed to us, and we understand what it has to teach us, we have power over the problem, and we can apply the principles we've learned to it and new situations. We don't need to be troubled by that particular lesson in the future.

The issue for many people is that they get caught up in the situation. They're confused by the experience of being a part of the problem. They blame other people and circumstances rather than figuring out how to correct the problem in their thinking.

Some time ago, a woman came to see me about a problem she was having with her family. This woman had many "shoulds" for both her husband and her two teenage sons. You'll learn more about the dangers of "shoulding" in just a bit, but in this person's situation, she wanted her husband and sons to behave in definite ways and think the way she did. She became frightened when her husband began spending less and less time at home, and her sons began getting into trouble in school. She dragged all three of them into my office to be "straightened out."

This woman was caught up in having her family resist and move away from her. Her lesson to learn was to forget about finding new ways to bring them under her control but to see that, whenever she tried to control those she loved, she invited resistance and drove them away. The lesson is that judgment and control are not the qualities you probably want to display, because they'll always invite negative results. Once she could see the meaning, she learned the lesson, she became less controlling, and the problem dissolved.

If there's a problem in your life, be assured that it's there for your growth and edification. Problems arise because we fail to see the truth of how the universe operates. We have misconceptions that require correction. Our thinking is the problem.

Jesus said, "Ye shall know them by their fruits." This means that you will know the truth by the result. If things aren't going well, or if you're angry, unloved, or living in poverty, there are truths about life to understand.

Our progress in life clearly depends on how we think. Our progression to a better, more fulfilling life, filled with the results we want, depends on expanding our "knowingness." Expanding knowingness is different from knowledge. Although doing all we can to learn everything we can helps, developing knowingness adds a patina of richness to our experiences.

To better understand, let's look at a simple analogy. An architect designs a spacious room and installs the windows at just the right places to bring the outdoor view into the room. The mechanics of the building and the dimensions of the room might be made up of formulas that guarantee spaciousness and balance. Being in the room might be a pleasant experience, or the room might need to have its edges softened to be more enjoyable. So, one who is gifted with the ability to choose and arrange furnishings brings together the structure and space to make it a unique setting. The mechanics can only go so far; then creativity and style are expressed to reflect originality.

Similarly, lessons can do the same for us. We can live by the rules, regulations, and formulas for success that are available to anyone who seeks today's answers. This is one of our options. A better and a more progressive way is to consciously choose the concept that the challenges and the lessons we can learn from them came into our life to tutor us. We can then reflect the growth and experience of learning the lesson and grow into the next level of character and originality.

Lessons are one of life's guarantees. If you think about them correctly, they are some of life's best gifts. They come to us one after another. As soon as we've completed one, we have another one to deal with. Each lesson brings us the gift of knowledge that living and learning provide. This knowingness is nurtured into greatness by even more lessons. As you read this, I'm certain that a lesson is present in your circumstances. It's waiting for your cooperation before it can give you the increase in awareness and understanding it has for you—an increase that will elevate you to the next level of your life.

The more lessons we have, the more we know. The more knowledge we have, the more options we have to exercise. You would think we would welcome and crave lessons for all the good they do. But often people avoid the next lesson by holding on to the present one. As each lesson is resolved, we move on to the next one with sharper skills, lighter hearts, and more creativity and energy.

We attract the lesson at the time we need to learn it.

The successful resolution of the lesson at hand guarantees the next lesson. Each lesson builds on the last. Once one grasps the importance and principle of lessons, momentum toward success is recognized.

A Case History About Lessons: Trillian's Story

This story demonstrates how lessons can help develop the power of knowing what you want and believing you can have it. It's about identifying the obstacles and maneuvering around them.

Trillian is a 7-year-old who lives in Eureka, California, with her father, Trevor. She's a bright and sensitive child who does well in school, and she has lots of friends. One Friday afternoon, she and her father went to a strip mall in nearby Humboldt, and Trillian discovered a keen pair of pink cowgirl boots. The moment she saw them she fell in love with them, and she had to have them. While still in the store, she asked her dad if he would buy them for her. She said, "Oh, Papa, I just have to have them. They've got *me* written all over them!"

Her dad said, "I'm sorry. I can't afford to buy you the cowgirl boots because we're short on money this month, and they're a luxury item. Besides, I'm buying you the braces you need for your pretty smile. But you could buy them for yourself with the money you have in savings."

Trillian's response was: "I know I have money in my savings account, but that was from Grandma at Christmas, and I don't want to spend it. I want to keep saving it. I'll just have to come up with a way to get those pink cowgirl boots! They are so *me*."

The next morning was a Saturday, and Trillian woke up her dad and said, "I've figured out a way to get those pink boots! I'm having a yard sale! You know I have a lot of toys and stuffed animals and some clothes I don't need anymore. There are lots of kids around here who would really like to have some of that stuff. They have money, and they get allowances, so I'm having my sale today. I'm going to put a blanket on the ground in the front yard and put my things out on the blanket. Then customers will come and give me money so I can get those pink boots."

Trillian put her plan into action and was busy most of the day setting up her sale and taking in her proceeds. There was a lot of bargaining going on, as well as some strong salesmanship, while she liquidated her collection. Her sensitive nature came into play when her customers' desire for one of her items was greater than their money, so she let a lot of things go for less than the value she had put on them. At the end of the day, she had raised enough money to buy the pink cowgirl boots, and she had created a vacuum by making room in her closet, and in her life, for more good.

That Saturday evening at dinner, she asked her dad if he would take her back to the strip mall in Humboldt the next day so she could purchase the boots. He explained that he wasn't available to take her then but that he could take her the next week. Eager to have the boots, resourceful little Trillian went back to the drawing board of her mind for Plan B.

At bedtime, she approached her dad and explained that she'd struck up a deal with Julie, her next-door neighbor. The deal went something like this: "Julie can take me to Humboldt tomorrow so I can get my boots. Is it okay if she takes me? And because she's going to help me, I promised her I would babysit one hour for her while she goes to the store. So, can I go?"

Trevor said yes.

Sunday morning arrived, off to the store Trillian, Julie, and Julie's baby went, and Trillian put her money on the counter to pay for the boots. She had negotiated her way to her desired results by turning a field of obstacles into a field of dreams. Rather than concentrate on the limitations the lesson was presenting, she focused on her abilities, created a way to have what she wanted, and learned a great lesson about herself.

Hold on a second; it gets better. Much to Trillian's surprise, the clerk said, "You've given me too much money." As it turned out, the boots had just gone on sale, and Trillian had money coming back. Thrilled, Trillian put on her new pink cowgirl boots and got in Julie's car.

This story demonstrates the power we all have (no matter how old we are) to claim what we want, believe that we can have it, become open and receptive to the ideas and the kinds of thinking we need to accomplish to make it happen, and then follow up on the guidance and direction those ideas give us. I think it's possible to have the vision, to develop the belief, to navigate through obstacles in our thinking, to take whatever action is required, to learn the lesson, and to do the work that needs to be done to reach our goals. After following these guidelines, we are rewarded with results that surpass our expectations. Not only did Trillian claim and work for what she wanted, she also recycled and cleared out the old to make way for the new. Her lesson helped her to learn how powerful she could be, and while she was learning it she also made a profit!

This brings up a key point: A lesson is repeated until learned. Simply put, if we don't choose to get the gift the lesson has for us, it repeats itself until we finally accept the truth about what we need to know to develop our consciousness. If we refuse to learn the lesson, the people, places, and circumstances might change, but the lesson stays the same and keeps reappearing until we accept its gift of growth and master it.

When avoidance seems like an option in dealing with our lessons, we might want to remember that the names and faces change, but the lesson remains the same until learned. For example, we all know people who repeatedly attract destructive relationships into their lives. They often believe that if they can get the "problem person" out of their lives or change his or her personality, everything will be fine. It's the nagging parent, or the unloving husband, or the rebellious child. The belief is that if only these people would change, life would be better. But the truth is that each of us has to look at what we are thinking, feeling, and doing that attracts difficult people into our lives.

You can tell that your consciousness is being enlightened by your lessons when you show more confidence, success, and prosperity. On the other hand, if you're a walking chart of battle scars of unfortunate circumstances or events, perhaps you're repeatedly having the experience without understanding the lesson. You grow through the experience of learning the lesson. Then, as you experience the realization that you've extracted what the lesson has to teach you, you throw away the experience and keep the lesson.

How many people do you know who go on and on about some difficult time in their life? They rehash what happened and how it held them back. In fact, it's still holding them back, because they're still focusing on the experience, instead of learning the lesson and being on their way. If you're back in the past where you were hurt, thinking of the unfair things that happened to you, your focus on the experience of how awful it was will keep you from figuring out what you need to do to make your life better now. If you're living in the past, you're not going to resolve the problem. Many of us think that if we don't remind others of what we've been through, they won't be able to know that we hurt and healed. More likely, however, they're sick and tired of hearing our victim stories. When we think of ourselves as being victimized—and, even worse, go on and on about it to anyone who'll listen—it's a sure sign we're missing the lesson life is offering us. People would be better off to be known by what they have learned from their lessons rather than the grueling growth they had to go through to get there. Through our lessons and the growth that promotes enlightenment, we develop consciousness. Rather than expressing the consciousness of one who's going through something awful, it's better to come off as one who's been there, who grew, and who now has something to reflect and contribute.

When we seem pressured by our lesson, the pressure often is interpreted as a pressure of time. We think: "Where would I be had this intrusion not set me back?" To see the lesson as friend instead of foe, one concept to develop is that we all have plenty of quality time to develop our thinking and consciousness. If we all spent a little more time figuring out the meaning of our problems, we wouldn't be wasting time with the fussing, fighting, and blaming that plagues human existence.

> *You cannot dream yourself into a character; you must hammer and forge yourself one.*
>
> ~ Henry David Thoreau (1817–1862), philosopher and poet

Many of us are in too big a hurry. We must choose to invest quality time and skill in dealing with our lessons to achieve peace of mind. This creates more time—time to enjoy demonstrating the consciousness we've formed and the results or fruits that it will attract.

Consciousness is our level of thinking. We could all reflect more consciousness if our thinking was more elevated. It's developed by our lessons—those helpers in our lives that are repeated until learned, and that provide growth and develop character. The greatest hope for any one of us is that our level of being conscious will expand through our lessons, and eventually we'll achieve an enlightened understanding. Let's welcome our life lessons with the anticipation that with them comes more awareness of how life is an unfolding adventure and an opportunity for us to increase our capacity to think and rethink our options.

Common Misconceptions Leading to Lessons

Two common flaws in thinking cause many problems that humans deal with. First, there is the belief in "shoulds." Whenever we hear the word *should* come out of our mouths, we know we're headed for trouble. The second idea that generally results in a lesson is the idea that our problems come about as a result of other people and circumstances rather than from our minds. Let's explore these two common misconceptions in detail.

Misconception #1: There are "shoulds" for ourselves and others.

Often we are frustrated while experiencing a lesson, because we haven't made appropriate choices. There's a negative term called *shoulding*—the habit we all have of saying "I should do this. I should do that." Whenever we hear ourselves "shoulding," we're not aware of what's appropriate. When we say "I should do this," there is a sense of not choosing or wanting to do what we "should" do. When we say "I should," it takes away the delight of doing something because we want to.

Whenever we hear ourselves saying "should," we need to stop and ask: "Am I thinking I'm being forced to do this? Maybe this thinking isn't appropriate, and I need to look at this situation to determine if it's one of my priorities." If we choose an action, we also need the ability to see the results that doing it wholeheartedly will bring. As we change channels from "I should" to "It's my choice," the process won't be working against us, but it will flow as our good is being realized.

Even if you've grown into a wise and aware adult, you can still sabotage yourself because you feel you should do something. When you feel that you're being forced into doing anything, it's human nature to stick out your lip and say: "I don't like this, because it's being forced on me." It might be a responsibility that you've lined up yourself, or one you might have accepted with the territory, but you still might retaliate, resent, and sabotage yourself.

Recalling the "genie appearance" described in Chapter 3,

reflect on your genie's offer and what you decided you really want from this lifetime. Once you can see the desired outcome, instead of beating yourself up and procrastinating, you can be in the process of getting there.

A flaw in thinking that causes even more problems for us than our shoulds for ourselves is our shoulds for other people. When we decide we know more about how other people should think or behave than they do, we are condemning, judging, and blaming. We create expectations that are bound to frustrate and disappoint. The more we try to force others to do things they don't want to do, the more they'll resist us. They will sabotage us, fight with us, undermine our efforts, and eventually reject us.

How often have you heard people say the following?

"She should meet my needs."

"He should be more understanding."

"She should show me more respect."

"He should love and support me."

It's common to hear people say over and over that their significant others should think, feel, and behave the way the person thinks they should. The fact is, they can't and won't, and if you hang onto your shoulds, you'll continually feel frustration, anger, and disappointment. These uncomfortable feelings will be the direct result of your *should thinking*. Those feelings will motivate you to behave in ways that are against your best interest. That behavior will most likely result in a negative life experience.

When you hear yourself say "I should," "he should," or "she should," catch yourself. Shoulding is a flaw in thinking that will bring about a negative lesson.

Misconception #2: Life's difficulties come from outside us rather than from our minds.

Some of us are stuck with lifelong situations, and, if we're not careful, our retaliation and resentment will stop us dead in our tracks. We won't be dead as in dead and buried, but we will vegetate because of our inertia, our anger, our frustrations, and our inability to determine what's appropriate.

You might have some situation or condition that's going to be with you your whole life. It could appear to be a handicap. It could be a flaw in your appearance or in a member of your family. It could be a situation that might label you, but you can consider it something that you work with and still create a successful life in spite of it. I knew a quite-successful woman whose husband was uncomfortable to be around. She loved him, she saw his (very) hidden qualities, she apologized for his lacks, and she went on to live the life and develop the success she wanted. Knowing that a similar situation is going to be with you for some time, you can work as productively as you can with the given set of circumstances. We've all heard stories of people who inspire others because they've turned an illness or handicap into an opportunity for growth. Instead of thinking of themselves as victims, they've actually made more of their lives than they might have without their particular challenge.

You have the option of thinking of yourself as a victim, or you can approach your particular challenge with the character, the special creativity, and the warmth and charm that only you can give to the situation that plagues you. You have the opportunity to turn the problem into your finest hour as you move through the lesson.

More than likely, what seems to be something you'll always be stuck with—an income or health level or something negative in all your relationships that just doesn't seem to go away—needs be handled appropriately for you to move ahead. With a shift in attitude, the situation can be turned into an opportunity for growth. You must take responsibility for creating this shift.

Naturally, if a tragedy occurs in your life, you will be hurt and you will grieve. If, however, you remain angry or disappointed by your lot in life year after year, this positive resolution can't happen. Know that you are too positive a thinker to be stuck with an unpleasant lifetime situation.

An important truth about being human is that we can't control other people, and we can't control life circumstances. What we *can* control is our thinking. We have control over how we choose to think about the various challenges life offers. It's not what happens to us but how we choose to think about what happens to us that determines our feelings, behavior, and experiences. We can see ourselves as victims, or we can look at each challenge—each lesson—as an opportunity for growth.

Practical Steps for Dealing with Lessons

> *The gem cannot be polished without friction, nor a man perfected without trials.*
>
> ~ Chinese proverb

The only way to have peace of mind is to discipline our minds. Let's next look at the "how to" steps for dealing with lessons. First, look at your challenges, and identify each one. (If you're like most people, there is probably more than one.) Then identify what makes you uncomfortable about the challenge or difficulty. You might want to make a list on paper so you can see it more clearly. Sometimes putting things in writing helps us to focus on them. Confining them to paper condenses the "massiveness" that they've had in our thoughts and makes them more manageable.

List your challenges, and identify the difficulty.

> Identify your thinking about your challenges. Ask yourself if you should reposition your thinking and claim ownership of the challenge and the result you desire. Exercise

your authority over the challenge and your thinking, and realize that you are happening to the challenge, rather than the challenge happening to you.

To help adjust your thinking, answer these questions.

What is this lesson or challenge showing me I need to learn?

Which qualities that I already possess can this opportunity strengthen?

What will be the result of my *growing* through this, rather than just *going* through this?

Have I had similar experiences? If so, what did I learn to help me with this one? What did I avoid learning in the past that I need to learn now?

When I think about my problem, what "shoulds" do I have for myself?

When I think about my problem, do I have "shoulds" for others? Am I trying to control someone else?

Am I blaming other people and circumstances for my problem?

Adjust your thinking and identify the lesson you choose to learn from the challenge.

Formulate your lesson in words. Focus on new ways to think about the problem so that it becomes a challenge. From this adjustment in thinking, new feelings will emerge. Identify new behaviors that will help you rather than contribute to the problem.

Keep the lesson, and throw away the experience.

The third step is to separate the experience from the lesson. After you've learned what the lesson has to teach, forget about all the "who did what to whom" memories, and move ahead in your life.

Separating the experience from the lesson also takes away the hurt and bad feelings. It relieves the harmful effects of blame and empowers you with energy and vision to focus on (1) what needs to be accomplished, (2) how to accomplish it, and (3) how to increase in awareness and consciousness.

Write a list of affirmations to change the problem thinking and to discipline your mind.

Changing a lifetime of thinking a certain way takes time and discipline. The most practical way of changing your thinking is to affirm statements of your productive new thoughts. Write statements of how you want to think about yourself and your situation. Such statements might be: "I can finish that project today," or "I can talk with my boss without being afraid," or "I can pass that adult education class." Read them every day. Post them where you will see them frequently. Record them onto a CD, and play them when you're riding in your car. Through effort and repetition, your new ideas will become second nature.

Next, let's see how you can implement this formula in your life.

I'd like you to meet someone I'll call Gary. Gary isn't a real person, but he is a good representation of many people I've worked with over the past decades. At this point in his life, Gary has lived a rather successful life, his needs are generally met, and he has a family, a home, and a good job. He is loved and respected, and he considers his life mostly good. Actually, Gary isn't satisfied, because he'd like for life to be better than good, and somehow he knows it's not going to get that way without his involvement. He feels frustrated because he doesn't know exactly what to do. One day he reads the guidelines I've just given you and decides to give it a try. He sits down with pad and paper, and under "List your challenges and identify the difficulty," Gary starts to write. His writing, spurred by a mixture of frustration and inspiration, starts to resemble a three- or four-page letter. He questions why he's writing so much, but, because he's on a roll, he just lets it all out. He comes to the end, and then he reads and rereads his outpouring. By the third time, he starts to read between the lines, and he can begin to see patterns.

On fresh paper, Gary jots down random words and phrases from his description of his challenges and starts to create a list of difficulties. On his list he states that he's overloaded at work and at home, as well as with the demands he places on himself. Furthermore, although he's making headway, he doesn't receive the recognition for which he feels worthy.

Gary has just done something wonderful for his thinking. He's in the process of opening a door to a new room in the mansion of his mind. Fine-tuning his list, he can easily see that his lesson is a reflection of his thinking. In fact, he sees that his life reflects his thinking: "There's too much to do, not enough time, and no appreciation."

He catches his concept in midair as he moves on to the next step: "Adjust your thinking, and identify the lesson you choose to learn from the challenge." He can see the step he needs to take to become a person who manages his thinking and his life so that he will have plenty of time, plenty to do (effectively), and appropriate recognition. Something inside him is saying: "This is your chance, your answer, your breakthrough."

Often, these "break through your thinking" moments offer much clarity. Gary might see that, as a child, he grew up in an environment that supported the ideas that there is too much to do and not enough time, and that the effort he applies won't be appreciated. His parents were demanding and critical, and they rarely complimented his efforts. As a young adult, he chose to involve himself with situations that reflected the emotional climate in which he grew up. Now, as an adult, he sees that he continues to perpetuate this old, familiar script.

He also becomes aware that his old way of thinking was filled with "shoulds," such as "I should be able to accomplish more" and "Other people should appreciate me." He can also see that he was falling into the trap of blaming circumstances rather than knowing his life difficulty came from his mind. He sees that his thinking incorporated both of the misconceptions leading to lessons.

As Gary grasps this new concept, he can discipline his thinking to throw away his past experiences and take a giant step into a positive future. In this step of throwing away the experience, Gary forgives those people and experiences he's been blaming. He accepts the responsibility for his thinking. He is preparing himself to throw away the experience and keep the lesson.

He's now ready to focus on what he needs to accomplish in his thinking and how he'll accomplish it. He builds an affirmation list to guide his thinking toward the results he desires. Gary writes, and then says aloud: "I have plenty of time. There's enough time to do all I need to do. I'll choose and prioritize my work, and my efforts and effectiveness will be noticed."

Already he feels the momentum of being drawn to more happiness, success, and prosperity. There is no longer the desire to blame, settle the score, or revisit the experience.

Because Gary knows that there's more ahead in life and more to become, he can eventually forgive and release the past, including all who were involved. He forgives himself for not getting this done sooner and then steps into motion to implement his breakthrough concept.

At this point his work has just begun, and he'll need to use his new thoughts every waking moment of each new day. He'll want to affirm aloud his new ideas several times a day. He could even use a CD or an app on his phone, put his affirmation list on his bathroom mirror, and carry it in his shirt pocket. The more diligence with which he applies these ideas, the faster the results will come.

In his relationships and in his workplace, "how it was" will often appear and can be a reminder each day to keep his thinking on the new level. Almost instantly, he'll feel new feelings about his life, his future, his time, and his abilities, and he'll see tangible results in these areas. Best of all, he'll receive tangible support from those around him, and he'll be recognized as a hero who conquered his own dragon or sea monster by taking charge and upgrading his thinking about the experiences of his life and the lessons they taught him.

There will be lessons for each one of us. These lessons will be repeated until learned. The way to achieve an enlightened consciousness is to learn the meaning of the problem, keeping the lesson and throwing away the experience. Next, discipline your mind to accept the new ideas by affirming the truth on a daily basis. Then expect the result to be a new level of consciousness, which will affect your life first as thoughts, then feelings, then behavior, and finally as life experience.

Your Map to "I'll Do the Work, Let Go of the Experience, and Keep the Lesson"

Take responsibility for your thinking and your memory. See the experiences you've had as opportunities for learning. Remember what you've learned. Forget the details of how you got here.

Avoid shoulding. Change "I should" to "It's my choice to _____."

See yourself as the curator of your own museum. Display your collection of treasures that you collected on your journey.

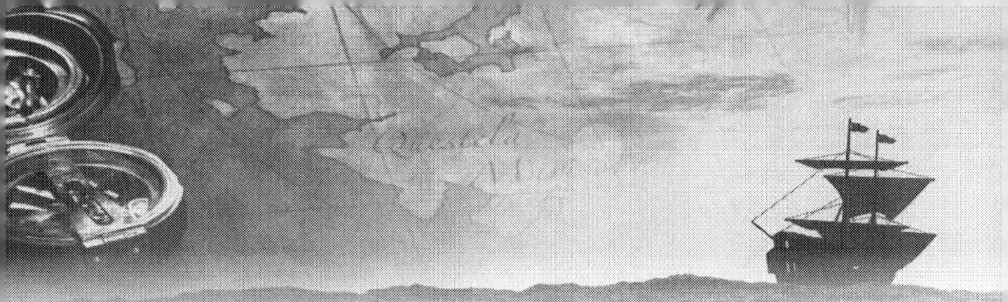

Chapter 11

Celebrate: Reach Your Goal

The reward of a thing well done is to have done it.
~ Ralph Waldo Emerson (1803–1882),
American essayist, lecturer, and poet

REACHING your goal and crossing the finish line is cause for a celebration. It's vital to know, once you've arrived, what you'll do to reward yourself for making the accomplishment and doing all it took to get to this point. It's also important to imagine what treasures you'll bring back from your terra incognita experience to furnish your life and bring you the reward you deserve for being such a daring explorer who forged through the unknown and expanded consciousness. Also, it's important to think ahead and to speculate how your return to the Harbor of Thinking will look and feel. What changes do you think you'll notice in your awareness of who you are and how you feel? What goals will you set for yourself in the future? When will you launch into your next exploration to the unknown?

In the chapter on setting goals and putting them in writing, you learned the importance of vividly visualizing the end result and having a clear picture of what your success will look like.

Time, energy, imagination, and creativity need to be invested into this vision, and, once it's established, you need to step into it, own it, and let it fuel you with energy and persistence to reach your goal. Interruptions, frustrations, and setbacks will come, but your vision of a successful completion of your goal and how you'll celebrate it will keep you on track and help you arrive at the finish line, cross it, and then celebrate your victory just as you imagined.

Celebrating your success is a well-deserved way to reward yourself for surviving your trek through all you had to do, sacrifice, and become to get to where you are. Part of the celebration needs to include a time of reflection on the adventures you had and how far you've progressed, the things you learned about yourself, the parts of you that were traded in for the new you, and the changes and increased consciousness you've created, and how they'll influence your future.

I know a woman who dramatically changed her appearance because of the work she did on upgrading her attitude, thinking, and health. She wanted her outer appearance to match her new level of living, so she visualized a new wardrobe, and her need, desire, and vision took her on a journey through her unknown. She could clearly see what she wanted, and she forged through feelings of limitation and unworthiness, which helped her change her thinking and create a clear goal. She had the interest and belief, and she claimed what she wanted, put her claim in writing, and, at a turtle's pace, reached her goal.

On her way to success, she had a garage sale, took her nicest clothing to an exclusive women's resale shop, and gave clothing to friends and to the needy. Cash rolled in to pay for her dream, and through the Law of Attraction and the Law of Magnetism she found an energetic saleswoman at a department store who sold her basic outfits she could mix and match, and gave her great ideas for accessorizing them to create dozens of new looks. She arrived at her goal, and her celebration was earned after doing all the work she had to do on her perceptions of whom she thought she was and what that person deserved and should look like. A metamorphosis took place, and, not only did she create a new outer appearance, but the radiance of who she had become in the process shone through.

Now, we're getting to the best part. After reaching her goal and feeling great about what she accomplished, how generous she had been, and how much enjoyment she anticipated about sharing her new look and consciousness with her future, she found that, while she'd been away on her journey, when she returned everything had changed—or so it seemed. Her appearance had changed from doughty to delightful, and she was different enough that other people could see this. Her loyalty and devotion to her career were also recognized for the first time in what seemed a very long time. She received a raise in pay and recognition for her efforts.

The universe will reward you for taking risks on its behalf.

~ Shakti Gawain (b. 1948),
author of books on personal development

Just think of our heroic explorers and the giants whose shoulders we visualized standing on in the beginning phases of their great journeys. They had the urge to go, and they believed they would find and claim honor and riches. They knew it would require stamina and fortitude and that they would return, like conquering victors, to accept their rewards and accolades. Surely their vision of a successful return and celebration aided their success.

I've told you about the transformation I undertook more recently, but one of my most challenging efforts to create successes and reach a goal occurred when I claimed a goal of attending college. Graduating from college was a requirement for my career, and I would be the first person in my family to do so. Associated with this goal was the vivid picture of the celebration I would enjoy after accepting my diploma in the traditional cap and gown. As I claimed this goal and pictured the celebration at the end, little did I know of the obstacles and victories that awaited.

In early August I would finish my four-year contract with the United States Navy. I made the appointment to take the Scholastic Assessment Test (SAT; the test for college admission). The timing of the test was tight; I would get the results just days before the deadline to enroll for college.

I had been working at the church I had found during my days in the Navy. During that time of gathering experience to become a minister and learning about church work, I had the glamorous job of assisting the minister on Sunday mornings and at midweek worship services, and the unglamorous job of sexton, Sunday bulletin printer, errand runner, and office staffer. Best of all, I was the sponsor of the youth group. This energetic group of high school–aged young people became my congregation, and from them I learned how I would develop my own style of ministry while I learned about teaching, keeping the group awake and motivated, fundraising, social dynamics, the need for fun, and how to deal with various personalities and emotions.

I was enrolled in summer seminary classes, but I was so determined to make college life the next chapter of my life that on several occasions I went to the college to get a feel for my future. I explored the campus and found the library, the English and science departments, the cafeteria, and the Quad, where bulletin boards, concerts, and demonstrations were the focal point of student life. I even took note of how everyone dressed. Completely caught up in my goal, I could see my bright future before me, full of promise and excitement.

When I returned from summer seminary classes in Kansas City, Missouri, I went to the site where I had taken the SAT to see my score that had been posted. Much to my dismay, I couldn't find it anywhere on the published list. When I asked how my name could have been left off, I was informed that the lowest scores didn't make it onto the list and weren't posted. Not only was my name not on the list of results, but, worst of all, I wouldn't be going to college in the fall. The "master plan" for my life suffered a bad blow. It was such an embarrassing predicament that I couldn't tell anyone, and I didn't know what to do.

I shared my defeat with my minister and mentor, who had a great idea. He reminded me that Genevieve, an elderly woman in our church family, was a retired school principal, and perhaps she might have some ideas. Genevieve and I met, and she was willing to help me acquire the education I needed to successfully pass the next SAT.

During elementary school I was an outgoing and fun-loving child, but not the best student. No one knew what attention deficit disorder was in the late '40s and early '50s; all I knew was that I found it hard to stay focused in class, and my attention was often diverted by my vivid imagination and wandering mind. When I took tests I gave answers, but they weren't the answers the teachers wanted. I tried very hard to keep up, but I realized that, to protect myself from criticism at making barely passing grades, I'd have to make up for it in other areas. I displayed artistic abilities, creating great drawings, posters, and salt maps, and I was really good at oral reports. I was also funny. These two qualities got me past the absence of passing test scores. Perhaps the teachers saw my winning personality, eagerness to please, and artwork as reasons to move me to the next grade. I was passed from grade to grade, but I entered each school year with less and less education. I guess I was "street smart" but not "test smart."

Genevieve gave me an evaluation test, and the results were devastating. Perhaps there was a chance that I could enter college someday, but first we had a lot of work to do. My income came from the work I did at the church. Thanks to the congregation's belief in my potential and their generous support for my education, I was able to pay Genevieve for her tutoring and start working on gathering the knowledge to get the highest score possible on the next SAT.

She began by saying: "You aren't stupid, you're a fine young man, and you have a good vocabulary and great people skills. Everyone likes you, and you're a natural for the ministry. It's that along the way, you didn't acquire the skills for passing testing." She explained that the testing she and I had done would give us a good idea of my grade level, and we'd move upward from that point. I was eagerly hoping that I had tested at the ninth- or 10th-grade level. I never felt lower than when she announced, "We need to build a strong foundation for learning, so we'll be beginning at the third grade."

Third grade? That would take forever! But there was no choice; I had to take the SAT to gain admission to college. I went through all the steps of procrastination, denial, rejection, and giving up, only to find that my goal was stronger. I got back in focus with my ultimate goal—to graduate from college and become an ordained minister—and mustered up the determination to go to school, starting at the third grade, with Genevieve every afternoon after completing my duties at the church. I knew the importance of setting goals, and this goal was to get the learning I had missed the first time around. I set the goal, and I vividly saw myself celebrating by taking my tutor and mentor to lunch.

The hours of study and development I spent with Genevieve were invaluable. Thanks to her patience and persistence, I slowly progressed through each grade. At the end of each grade I would be tested to see if I had learned everything I needed to know to move on to the next grade. I flew through third grade, but there was much more to absorb in each following grade. Yet I was on my way to graduating from high school for the second time. I have a vivid memory of heading to a dance club on a Friday night, where other young adults would be dancing and drinking and hopefully getting a phone number on a napkin. I remember thinking: "Tonight I'm going to celebrate! I just graduated from fifth grade!" As I entered the club, I realized how far I had to go; the club was filled with college students who had already qualified for college and were way ahead of me.

Over the next several months I continued to work at the church. I was also studying the philosophy of Unity and working hard to absorb its teaching. The Truth principles, as they're known, were anchors that held me in place and would later be the foundation for the career ministry that lay ahead for me. No one knew I was working my way through elementary school or that I was undergoing all the experiences that demanded a change in my identity.

Finally "graduation day" arrived, and Genevieve assured me that she believed I had earned the right to be retested. Based on my test results and hard work with her, she was confident that I would make the required passing score. I prayed hard to get a score that would get me into junior college, even if it meant I'd have to take remedial math and English. The long-awaited test day came, and I completed the testing and waited what seemed months for the results. When I went to the testing site and looked up my name, I was surprised and delighted to see that I had good scores and that my scores had qualified me for enrollment into college classes, which meant that I didn't have to take any remedial classes. It was a pleasure to realize this goal, and I celebrated just as I had envisioned: by taking my guests to my graduation celebration. My guests were Genevieve; my mentor, Reverend Robert Stevens; and a girl I was sweet on. The day after I enrolled, we all enjoyed lunch at the International House of Pancakes. A splendid time was had by all, and, after another session of seminary summer school, I returned to San Diego to attend Mesa College.

Reaching this goal and celebrating my success were the beginning of the launch to set and reach new goals, with expectations for celebration upon their completion. I had come full circle. I started from the Harbor of Thought on my way to discoveries I would make on my "I'll of Creativity, Attraction, and Choice." I slayed my monsters of disbelief and disinterest, I set my goals and put them in writing, I persisted at a tortoise pace to attract help I had never expected, I reached my goal, and then I celebrated my success just as I had pictured doing.

Your Map to "I'll Celebrate"

Put the cherry on top of your goal by knowing that the effort you put into it deserves recognition. Vividly visualize yourself as a success, worthy of celebrating.

See the celebration. Imagine the location and the guest list, and see yourself thanking all those who helped and supported you along the way.

Vividly see yourself returning to what was your old world with all the loot you gathered on your journey: higher esteem, deeper faith in yourself and your abilities, a new strong and successful presence, and a spirited sense of going back for more.

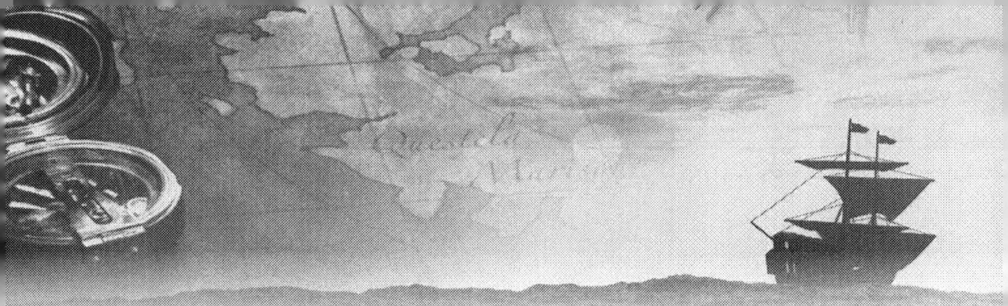

Chapter 12

Are You Ready to Go Back for More?

A hero is no braver than an ordinary man, but he is braver five minutes longer.

~ Ralph Waldo Emerson (1803–1882),
American essayist, lecturer, and poet

I'D like to share how I developed the basic concept of this book. Every time I apply this concept, it takes me forward and keeps me going back for more. I believe it makes me an expert.

It all started with an epiphany. An epiphany is a moment of revelation and insight, a sudden, intuitive perception of, or insight into, the reality or essential meaning of something—usually ignited by some simple, commonplace occurrence or experience, such as that moment the morning of my 59th birthday, which led me to achieving my vision and goal by my 60th birthday. I had always applied and taught those principles in my ministry, but on that particular day I found a new enthusiasm for putting them to work on a higher level. During this time I developed a clear focus about what I wanted and needed to do. I found I had the interest and the belief in my goals, and I decided to "go for it." I continually reviewed my desired goals, which I had in writing, in the areas of family, health, prosperity, mind, career, relationships, and spirit.

I made the commitment to do it and to take the time necessary each day to do all I could do that day to reach my goal. I had committed myself to go at a turtle's pace, keeping my goals in front of me all the time.

I had begun my journey of self-discovery and was on my way to my own terra incognita. All the things I've written about in previous chapters came to me bit by bit. As I incorporated them into my plan of success, they became the fabric of this book.

I learned about the turtle's pace, and searching took me to Aesop's fables and more. This led to a flashing back to the memory of that moment in fifth grade when Miss Long called on me for the answer. I remembered it was terra incognita, and I realized that would be what I would call my unknown. That led me to think about the explorers, their adventures, and the loot that they brought back. With my wild imagination I developed these ideas, tested them, and proved that they work.

I learned about the Law of Magnetism on a new level when my oral hygienist introduced me to the world of competitive running. After that first half-marathon, I was in a new phase of my life and my health. The culmination came at my birthday party, when my guests said, "I understand you're running now, and it really shows." This was the claim to fame I had known would come from the effort I was applying to all my other goals.

The Mexican Riviera cruise led to another unexpected success. While on the cruise, I had my body fat tested for the first time and began the journey of learning about nutrition and nutritional supplements. That was in October, and in late December I found the same body-fat measuring device at the Double Eagle Spa in June Lake, California, on our Christmas ski vacation. I took the test again and noticed a reduction in fat and a gain in muscle. This left me grateful and delighted; I had proof that what I was doing at a tortoise pace was really working.

Because I was genuinely interested in being as fit as possible, I entered a "build a new body" contest. I purchased and started taking the contest sponsor's diet supplement. I took my "before" photos required by the contest. I worked out and ran diligently. At the end of six months, I sent my "after" photos that documented the results I'd manifested over the six-month period. I ended up as a finalist in the top 100 applicants, and received a special certificate and a gym bag filled with the supplement product I had been taking.

I was measured again in March and again in July on another cruise ship. My final measurement came in September, at the time of our regular fall vacation to see the brightly colored aspens in June Lake. Just weeks before my greatly anticipated 60th birthday party, I had created the fat-free, muscle-defined body I had wanted for decades. Most of all, I had tangible results that were beyond my wildest dreams.

In summary, here is your copy of the map I created that took me to the success I enjoyed then and am enjoying today. An ideal beginning would be to create the opportunity and invite an epiphany—a moment of insight and revelation. Clearly see your options and possibilities, and welcome the inspiration to see what you want to create. Go to your heart, go to your wish list, go to your to-do list, and, as Gary did in that case study, go to your frustrations. Gather up your dreams and goals. Then take these steps:

Discipline your power of thought. Remember: Your ability to think about something differently is the key to opening the door of discovery.

Cultivate the power of creativity. Know that it's up to you to create the results you desire and that you can. Remember: If you can think it, you can create it.

Know that your thoughts and creativity will help you clearly see what you want and attract whatever you need to succeed.

Once your thoughts activate the Law of Attraction, your catalog of beliefs and possibilities is on its way.

Look through your options and opportunities; be aware of what you'd like to demonstrate.

Investigate your feelings and emotions, and discover that you truly have the interest in acquiring what you want, and that you truly believe you can do the work required to have what you want. Slay the monsters of Lack of Interest and Lack of Belief.

Decide you will have what you want and that you'll do whatever is necessary to arrive at your goal.

Put your goals in writing. Plot your course, leaving room for spontaneous events and time to navigate and negotiate through challenges from your old world. Include a timetable and schedule of your goal's unfolding, and vividly describe your celebration.

Keep track of your success. Begin doing the work, advance at a steady but slow pace, and chart your progress. Watch your seeds grow.

Become magnetic; draw information, input, and serendipitous support that will point the way to success. Attract help and inspiration along the way.

Celebrate reaching your goal!

> *I think a hero is an ordinary individual who finds strength to persevere and endure in spite of overwhelming obstacles.*
>
> ~ Christopher Reeve (1952–2004),
> actor and founder of a spinal cord research center

In an effort to stimulate your desire for this opportunity of discovery, here are some things for you to think about.

SUPPLIES:

You'll need a vessel, a compass, big sails, an anchor, nourishment, room to bring back the treasures you'll collect, and an energetic crew.

ATTITUDES:

You'll need a sense of adventure, dreams to follow, interest, belief, and courage.

UNNECESSARY CARGO:

No shots or vaccinations are required. You won't need any luggage (you don't have to pack or unpack), or a passport with an unflattering photo. You don't need a map, because you know where you want to go. Besides, the way there has never been charted. Your desire to reach newer, higher levels will get you there. And don't even think about cancellation insurance!

WHAT YOU WILL DISCOVER:

Anticipate the wonder and adventure ahead. Here's a list that you'll encounter; develop and discover it, and it will keep you inspired. You'll find a new sense of energy, esteem, and personal power. While there will be conflict from your old world, you can't let that keep you back. You'll collect treasures and riches that will finance future plans and dreams.

One of your most important discoveries will be that you've created a new world, and you'll find that you've already moved into it. You have created a new world that has dimension and shape in exchange for the old, flat one.

WHAT YOU WILL BRING BACK FROM TERRA INCOGNITA:

You'll be sitting heavy in the water, loaded with an increased awareness, health, longevity, prosperity, esteem, a new level of success, and the power to leave your old world and enter your new world. Perhaps best of all, you'll have the opportunity to let your success inspire your family, friends, and coworkers.

Let me tell you how you can get there from where you are right now. You can do it! Remember the formula:

To start:

Know the power of thinking.
Remember that you create the results.
Your thoughts attract.
See what you want.
Be really interested and believe.

Decide you'll have it:

Put your goals in writing.
Build and create it carefully and slowly.
Become magnetic.
Progress as your seeds grow.

Celebrate!

Dolly Parton uses a touch of her Southern charm and wisdom as she sings in her hit song: "You better start givin', forgivin', knowin', showin' concern about where you're goin'; better start carin', sharin' and be willin' to make a better way. You gotta stop whinin' and cryin'; you better start livin' so you can create a new day you get to live in!"

So the next time you find yourself hanging on to the edge for dear life, awaken with the answer and become a success, and your world will give you approval and reward you for thinking from a higher perspective.

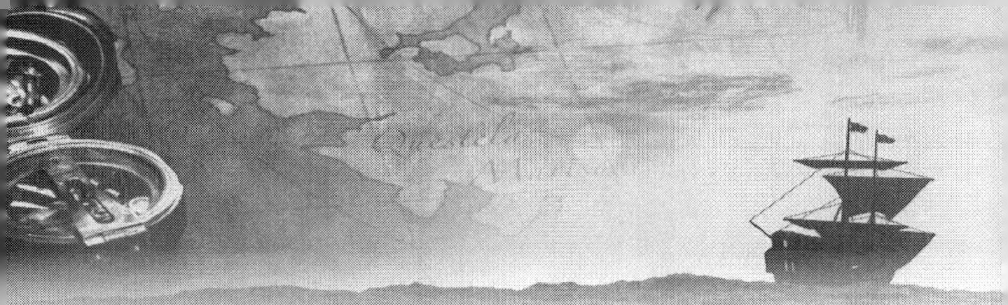

Chapter 13

The Principle of Having What You Want

It's our attitude at the beginning of a difficult task which, more than anything else, will affect its successful outcome.

~ William James (1842–1910), psychologist and philosopher

YOU can have what you want or something better. Over the years, I have learned that this principle works best if you put the needs of others ahead of your own. In this final chapter, I hope to convey how this principle has helped me reach the level of success I am so thankful to be enjoying at this time of my life.

There are times when you have to kedge yourself into position for success. There were times I had do this to get out of the doldrums of inactivity and position myself to benefit from the winds of change. *Kedging* is a technique for moving or turning a ship by using a relatively light anchor tow as a kedge. It can pull a boat out of shallow water when it has run aground, or there is no wind to push its sails. A dinghy is used to set an anchor, and then the boat is pulled toward the anchor. These steps are repeated until the boat is in water deep enough, or where there are conditions for wind, so that the boat and its crew can be on their way.

In a similar way, there are times when you have to take the situations in which you find yourself by the hand, pull yourself out of where you are, and pull yourself toward where you want to be. For you, kedging might involve ending a friendship with someone who constantly criticizes and complains. Or you might change your major in college to one that better fits your abilities and interests. Or you might move from your present job to one that pays less but is more fun. Perhaps my story of how I used this principle to create success in my life will be helpful in making this point come alive for you. When I started kedging my way to success, I didn't know what kedging was. I had never heard the term before. The only thing I knew was that, if I wanted to gain the results I so strongly desired, I would have to make it happen. Nothing was going to fall into my lap. I had to create an "if it is to be, it is up to me" attitude.

I reached my goal of becoming an ordained Unity minister. In fact, I was the youngest person that the Unity Ministerial School ever ordained. I had dreams of becoming a success at turning my ministry into a meaningful one that inspired people and changed lives. I wanted to be prosperous and have all my needs met. I wanted a future that included a successful career that was developed by hard work, creativity, service, and clever use of time and talent. I knew that simply waiting for it to happen wasn't going to make that success come along. At the same time, I believed that I was limited by my circumstances. I knew that in order to reach my goals, it was up to me to pull myself out of feelings of being stuck and pull myself into the stream of success. To find success, I would have to kedge my way toward it.

He who wishes to secure the good of others has already secured his own.

~ Confucius (551–479 BCE), philosopher

First, I had to define how I wanted my future to look and what it would contain. All during the time I was involved in church work, I had been studying successful ministries, and I had visions of helping people through a television ministry and community service. I also valued the principle of service, which included serving in the Association of Unity Ministers and our Southwest Region organization.

So I made the commitment and decision to get right to work and do all I could to be involved in these four areas: inspiring and helping people discover and reach their goals, developing a television ministry, serving my community, and being an active member of my local ministerial association. Making the decision started the wheels of progress moving. I was kedging myself out of the doldrums and setting my course for success while I determined what I wanted, regardless of how impossible it seemed. Little did I know the adventure I was creating for myself.

Things started to happen, and they happened quickly. I had a full-time ministry that was new for me, the people I served, and the community. I had many ambitious projects, including maintenance of the church building and the attached manse and fellowship hall. I had relationships to build, ministering to do, and a full schedule and calendar. Yet I knew that to have everything I wanted to be included in the grand total, I had to believe that I could create it if I devoted enough time to doing so, in addition to accomplishing all the other things on my list. So I got right to work, or perhaps I should say the work got right to me, because I believe our thoughts and desires become magnetic, and we attract the opportunities to have what we want.

In the area of community service, a member of my congregation invited me to attend a board meeting for the Heartland Creative Community Association (HCCA). The meeting was across the street from the church, which couldn't have been more convenient. As I was introduced to the board members, they explained the purpose of the association: to act as a nonprofit umbrella for organizations in the community that didn't have nonprofit status. These community organizations were being given donations, and their donors were hoping to receive tax write-offs.

One such group was made up of women who made lap robes for nursing homes. A fabric store was willing to donate cloth for their projects, but it wanted a tax deduction. These women didn't have the knowledge or time to apply to the State of California for nonprofit status, so finding the HCCA was an eminent blessing for their efforts and for the fabric store, too.

Another member of the association was just getting started and had plans to obtain nonprofit status. The support it received enabled it to use the HCCA tax number so it could give write-off privileges to a sponsor, which gave time for the application process at the state capitol. This was the kind of community service I desired to be part of, and volunteering to serve on the board of directors was an easy obligation. During the seven years I served this group, I learned the ins and outs of nonprofit protocol and state laws. As an association, we helped many groups get off the ground and make a difference in our community. My service resulted in gratitude for my giving back to the community. It also helped my self-image and my professional image and gave me knowledge about the nonprofit world, but, most of all, it prepared me to step into a situation that was going to make me extraordinarily happy.

The next area to conquer was to serve the organization in which my church and I were members. I became a volunteer board member of the Southwest Region of Unity Churches. Our duties were to attend board meetings in the Los Angeles area and support and encourage the 45 churches and ministers in our region, which included Southern California, Nevada, and Hawaii. We welcomed new ministries, helped our licensed teachers, offered to mediate disputes, attended celebrations and church openings, conducted an annual laymen's retreat, and managed the Region's funds. I worked my way up from member-at-large to secretary, treasurer, vice president, president, and finally regional representative, which was a position comparable bishop.

This time of service took years of many miles of travel and hours of laborious board meetings. Being selected by fellow ministers to be regional representative was a particular honor; their vote of confidence backed me up and demonstrated their belief in my abilities. My duties included necessary training to do troubleshooting, which enabled me to become an expert in handling disputes, and to attend official board meetings of the Association of Unity Churches at our world headquarters near Kansas City, Missouri. Eventually I was elected to the 12-member executive board, which is the leading decision- and direction-maker of the Unity Church ministries. Arriving at this position took years—years of meetings, mileage, and service. Little did I know how helpful this long process of becoming was going to be to my future.

I had no idea how to get started sharing my message with a television audience until a friend, Sherrie Ross, came in for counseling. She was a recent graduate of the Barbizon School of Modeling, and she had gone to this school to work in television and print modeling. She was extremely frustrated because she couldn't get into the business. I assured her that I would do all I could to help her realize her goal, and I confided in her that I, too, longed to gain experience before a television camera that I could later use for a television ministry. Together, we started working on our dreams.

I had recently taken pictures for our church newsletter with a photographer named Twyla. During our photo session, Twyla told me that she wanted to take more head shots and to photograph models. The three of us—Twyla, Sherrie, and I—put our heads together and came up with the idea of taking a pink piggybank into a local savings and loan, to serve as the background for Sherrie and me to pose as though we were about to break the bank with a shiny black hammer. Our idea was to create work for the three of us.

The photos turned out great. Sherrie and I marched into the best modeling and television production agency in San Diego and applied for work. There, we met Mary Crosby, owner and director of the Crosby Agency. Mary told us her stable of talent was completely full, and she wished us luck in our quest. Not taking no for an answer, Sherrie and I went to an ad agency next, and were pleased when the man in charge of talent gave us a chance at breaking into the business. It wasn't that simple, but after we made several visits to his office he said, "You two are just not going to give up! Come to my house on Saturday, bring lots of clothing to change into, and I'll take a lot of pictures of the two of you."

That Saturday we showed up, and he photographed us reading the newspaper in our pajamas, dressed in black tie and an evening gown for a night out on the town, by the pool in sneakers and T-shirts, and cooking in the kitchen. He told us he could use the photos for ads that would show us doing things that couples did. At the end of our photo shoot, much to our surprise he asked, "Where do I send the check?"

We were so surprised to find out we were getting paid that we didn't know what to say. Just as Sherrie was about to give him her address, a brilliant idea came to me, and I blurted out, "Send it to our agent, Mary Crosby."

Early the next week my phone rang. It was Mary Crosby, who said, "I have a check here, and I want to send you your part of it as soon as I take out my commission. By the way, who are you?"

I reminded her of our appointment a few weeks earlier and assured her that I would come to her office, pick up my check, and let her refresh her memory of me by seeing me in person.

That very afternoon, I accepted my check, and Mary asked, "What are you doing in the morning? I want to send you on a cattle call. The Purina Dog Food Corporation is making a commercial for television, and I need talent for it. Be in Presidio Park at 8 a.m."

Eight o'clock in the morning couldn't come fast enough! I was chosen to be in the commercial, I was given a dog, and filming began. We were dismissed when it became too warm and the sun too bright to continue filming. Later that day, Mary called again. This time she sounded desperate. "They've decided to add children to the shoot, and I need a handful of cute kids by eight o'clock in the morning! You have a Sunday school, right? Can you get me some kids quickly? They'll get paid, and they each get a big bag of dog food. Oh yeah—tell them to bring their dogs."

I immediately started making calls. By dusk, everyone had been contacted. Bright and early the next morning, we were filming. I was busy supervising the kids and dogs when the director's assistant informed me that because I was working so well with my troop of animals and humans, the director had dismissed the principal (industry talk for the star) and had chosen me to take his place. I had lines to learn and kids and dogs to direct, and I would be compensated and identified as a principal in a national commercial. The rest of the day went fine, and we wrapped everything up, put the kids, their moms, and the dogs into our cars, and returned to the church.

The next day, Mary sent me on a casting call. When I entered the room full of other men applying for the commercial, I felt extremely intimidated. I had never been in the company of such handsome, immaculately dressed and groomed men before. I distinctly remember thinking: "I might as well leave. These guys look so much sharper than I do that one of them is bound to get the job." One by one we were interviewed, and much to my amazement I received a call later that day informing me that I'd been chosen for the principal in another national television commercial. In my surprise I mentioned how much better looking the others were, and I was informed, "Yes, but you can talk."

Over the next eight months I was sent on eight casting calls, and I was selected for each of the commercials. My list of successes included Safeway Grocery Stores (playing a butcher), Home Federal Savings and Loan, and Turbo Lawn Mowers. One commercial was for Kentucky Fried Chicken, and I remember eating raw chicken because the fully cooked chicken photographed green. I have the pleasurable memory of going to my last audition and hearing one man who was trying out say to another: "We may as well leave; he gets every commercial he applies for."

This time in my life ended abruptly when there was a huge strike of film and television writers and other workers. The strike lasted 18 months, during which there was little to no commercial production. This was good for all of us who had residuals coming in but bad for those who wanted work. By the end of the strike I was involved in other projects and chose not to go back to making television commercials. There are times in our lives when one door closes because a new door is about to open.

> *The best way to find yourself is to lose yourself in the service of others.*
>
> ~ Mohandas K. Gandhi (1869–1948), political and ideological leader

And open one did! Years had passed while I was happily serving my community, serving the association of which I was a member, and gaining experience in front of television cameras. In addition to these investments into my career, I was managing the expansion of the church I had founded and was serving my congregation. There were Sunday sermons, midweek classes, memorial services, weddings, counseling, and the many social aspects of church work. I was busy and productive.

One day I received a call from a minister in distress, the Reverend Dale Batesole, who was asking for my help. He was calling me because I was the regional representative. He explained how a wealthy developer had approached him with a plan to give a gift of $150,000. This was to be given to the ministry he was serving in Palm Springs, California, for the purpose of creating a television ministry. The developer had the idea that a talk-show format featuring prominent movers and shakers would be his gift to the world, and that Dale was the best spokesperson for the job. Dale said that when he presented this idea to his board of directors they rejected the idea, saying that they liked things as they were and that a television ministry would change things too much. They also suggested that he go with the donor, and they terminated him on the spot. This led to his call to me.

Dale said he wanted to produce the television program and accept the $150,000, but he wasn't incorporated as a nonprofit organization and didn't have time to process an application before the donor went away.

My experience immediately started paying off. I assured my friend that he could immediately accept the gift by finding a minister friend who would allow him to come under his umbrella and borrow the other minister's nonprofit number until Dale could establish one of his own. I told him I knew how it was done, and had the contacts and paperwork he needed. He asked if he could come under the umbrella of my nonprofit corporation and borrow my number until he could establish one of his own. As soon as I agreed, he mentioned having seen me in the Safeway commercial. He not only invited me to be the first guest on his program, but he also invited me to give him advice on how best to present himself, because he'd never been on television.

All at once, what I had been giving out came back to me,

and it seemed that I had been set up for success. The television program *There Is a Way*, founded by the Reverend Dale Batesole, slowly grew to be a success. It was a full-time labor of love for Dale. His job included gathering guests, mailing them instructions and directions, and getting their subject matter from them as well as 10 questions for him to ask while their visit was taped. Five programs were taped in a two-day period each week at a television station in Palm Springs. Then the tapes were overnight-expressed to be aired on station KHJ in Los Angeles, which covered all of Southern California. A growing audience turned on the television five days a week from 7:30 to 8:00 a.m. to watch the program.

Dale interviewed authors, motivational speakers, experts in health, nutrition, and exercise, and every available Unity and Religious Science minster. Each guest brought a handout highlighting the topic, contact information, and information about his or her ministry or latest book. These handouts inspired viewers to mail a request for the handout and a donation to *There Is a Way*. Eventually these gifts met the expenses of creating the program. In return for their time, guests received exposure to a growing television audience all over Southern California. Minister guests reported healthy numbers of visitors on Sunday mornings, authors reported additional book sales, and motivational speakers told Dale of increased calls and interest. I was a frequent guest and among the most popular. (Popularity was measured by the number of viewer letter requests for a particular guest's handout and donations.)

After developing the program and putting a lot of hard work into its success, Dale decided to retire, and he invited me to take his place. I eagerly accepted and, after several months of coaching with him, became the producer, director, and host of what had become a stable television ministry with a viewership of over one million each week. During my time of service the program continued to increase in viewership and popularity. I will always be thankful for my eight years of presenting programs and that I was helpful in providing the opportunity for everyone who appeared as a guest to get out their message. I am confident that their presentations resulted in a wealth of ideas and inspiration to our viewers.

Life was incredibly busy. I had a lot to do to keep up with two ministries, travel between Palm Springs and San Diego each week, officiate at weddings each weekend, and supervise the construction of a new sanctuary at my church.

I wrote earlier about kedging yourself out of the doldrums, where there is no wind for your sails and shallow circumstances. I was acutely aware of what I wanted and what I needed to make happen to ensure the success I wanted in my career. I also knew that the results I desired weren't just going to come to me, but that I'd have to kedge myself to them. I'd have to pull myself out of where I was and how I was thinking about my situation. Having clear goals, putting them in writing, and doing all you can each day to take goals from dream to reality are the keys.

Although I had found the success I sought years before, things were about to become more wonderful than my wildest dreams could ever have imagined. One particular taping session changed everything. I was interviewing Dr. Virginia Foster. We had never met before, but I was familiar with her because I saw the audition tape her publicist had sent. She was a clinical psychologist practicing in Newport Beach, California. She was beautiful and bright. The 10 questions she submitted to become our script for the program were some of the sharpest I had ever received. To make things even better, she had generously delivered hundreds of copies of her latest book, *The Quest for Love and Money*, to be the handout for our viewers. I was excited to meet this first-time guest.

Because of the schedule, there wasn't a lot of time for visiting before taping began. After a brief introduction and review of our programming agenda with the three guests that day, taping began. The bright lights were on, the set was ready, and my first guest took his place. I asked the questions he had provided, and we taped the first program. Then, after changing into another shirt, tie, and jacket, I invited Dr. Foster to take her place. The theme song started, the announcer introduced the program, and I welcomed our viewers and introduced my next guest. I asked the scripted questions, and her answers were charming, polished, and intelligent. Then, without any notice, the bright lights suddenly went off, engulfing the set in darkness.

Over the loudspeaker in the production booth we heard, "We have a problem with camera one. We'll be right out to fix it. Just talk among yourselves, but don't talk about the program; it will lose its sizzle." So there, in the dim light, Virginia and I asked getting-to-know-you questions, quickly discovering that we both enjoyed country-western music, dancing, and skiing. We connected so strongly that Virginia said she would call me, and we'd go dancing or skiing. I only had time to blurt out "I'd like that" before a flood of bright light washed away what was becoming romantic lighting, and the voice from the booth announced, "Start where you left off." We picked up where we had been before the camera failure, neither of us missed a beat, we completed the program, and I thanked Virginia for her time and for her generous gift of her books. As she left the studio, I dashed into my dressing area for a new shirt, tie, and jacket.

That night I had a crash of emotions. It was my practice to add a little note to each donation thank-you letter to our loyal viewers. I signed hundreds of letters the two evenings I stayed in Palm Springs each week. That evening as I was signing, I realized what warm feelings I had had while visiting with Virginia and being in the company of such a bright and beautiful woman. Another realization that hit me like a ton of bricks was that I was so involved with my work and my two young sons that love and romance were vast, arid areas in my life. My thoughts kept going back to Virginia, and I wondered whether she would call.

The next day, after a busy morning of taping, I returned to my office to meet with the staff, review upcoming guests, and sign letters. I was told I had a call, and what I heard on the other end made me drop the phone. As I scrambled to get hold of the dangling receiver, I was thinking: "She called! It's Virginia!"

That call led to a ski weekend at June Lake, California, that began as a disaster but ended in love. I had assured Virginia I was an experienced skier. I had been skiing for two years by then, and I probably had put in about 40 full days on Mammoth Mountain. But when Virginia and I skied for the first time, my skiing was terrible. I must have been so focused on how beautiful she looked and how well she skied that I was out of touch with my skill. After falling a long way down a ski run, having a "garage sale" where everything flies off—gloves, skis, goggles, hat, you name it—and landing at the bottom of the run with a colorful trail of clothing and belongings strewn up the hill, I was helped to my feet by Virginia, who stepped out of her skis and climbed all the way up the run, gathering my stuff. She returned, helped to put me back together, and suggested we try a less-difficult hill.

My abilities returned as the day progressed, and by the end of the day I had redeemed my reputation. Nonetheless, I was lucky that the entertainment at the Red Lion Restaurant and Bar that evening was a country-western band. While the music played, Virginia and I two-stepped into each other's lives and hearts. Eight months later we were dancing at our wedding.

I'm always looking for events and circumstances to occur that I like to think of as signs that tell me I'm on the right track. I'll always think of one such event as miraculous. Shortly after the ski trip, Virginia took me to meet her parents. I was sure that she had told them all about me. After our meeting, Virginia's dad, Cleo, shared the experience with his best friend, John. He told John, "My daughter has fallen for this TV preacher, and I want the best for her, but I surely would like to know that he's sincere and on the up-and-up."

John asked, "On what television program or ministry does he appear?"

"The program is *There Is a Way,*" Cleo responded.

"Virginia's going to marry Arthur!" John said.

Cleo asked, "Do you know him?"

"No, I don't know him personally, but Marjorie and I start our day at 7:30 a.m. with his program every morning. We even saw him interview Virginia on it recently. He seems like a fine person to us."

This information couldn't have come to my future father-in-law in a better way or from a more reliable source. It paved the way for what was to become a very special friendship between Cleo and me.

It's a big world, and this appeared to be a sign that Virginia and I were on the right track. Little did I know when all this started that I was kedging myself to be in the best position to live a life of service to others. Those efforts became a life that yielded all the results I desired. I knew what I wanted, I put it in writing, and, although the desired results seemed quite far away, I did all I could (kedged) to reach them. Each of those hours of meeting with the community association, those miles of travel and meetings with the regional ministers, and the effort of going to those casting calls and working on the sets for television commercials resulted in my having what I wanted.

I offer this example as a suggestion that you, the reader, decide what you want. Put your goals in writing and do everything possible to pull yourself to your goal. Along the way, it's imperative that you do all you can to help those around you reach their goals, too. Look for signs along your way that will boost your efforts with nudges and insights that validate your goals and plans. Be careful that you assess these signs objectively. Your eagerness to succeed in a particular area could cause you to interpret them with a slant. Remember: You can have what you want if you help others get what they want, and often you have to pull yourself into your dream in spite of situations that seem beyond your control.

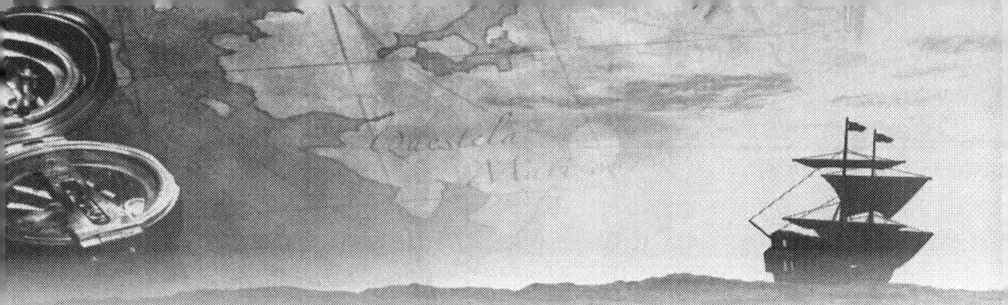

Conclusion: Your Maps of Discovery

THE content in this book has been about you making discoveries in terra incognita, bringing quality experiences and awareness back to your old world beliefs, and moving into the new level of success you desire. I trust the various true stories and individuals you have been introduced to have inspired you to go to your own terra incognita and make great discoveries. I am sure your journey will be exhilarating, scary, and challenging at times. And, I am equally positive your desire to create the best life you can live will stimulate all your talents and dreams, and empower you with the goals, stamina, and persistence you'll need. The results you can create will be so uplifting to yourself and those around you, and you'll return from your adventures to meet success, health, and prosperity beyond compare. I trust that this book has pointed the way for you to create your own stories and triumphs on the way to your terra incognita. Bon voyage!

Here is the path that you have been following through this book. It is also the path that will take you through your unknown and help you make the greatest discoveries for increasing and magnifying who you are and who you can become. Here are the maps to your success.

Your Map for Thinking

Begin by believing that your thinking is your internal guidance system and that it will move you to new heights.
Seek illuminating thoughts. This kind of thinking will spark ideas, and you will be inspired to action.
Expect results. You'll develop the awareness of what to do and how to develop the ability to do it.

Your Map to "I'll Use Creativity to Reach My Destination"

Develop an attitude of complete responsibility for your life.
Identify yourself as the responsible one for creating what you want.
Decide that you have the interest and belief that you can have what you want.
Be prepared to do the work required.
Anticipate the inspiration and delivery of your catalog of possibilities and beliefs.
Be prepared to put your goals in writing.
Develop the capacity to visualize the result and create a schedule for what you need to do.

Your Map to "I'll Accept Delivery of My Catalog of Possibilities and Beliefs"

Let empowered thinking and creativity stimulate the Law of Attraction.
Start anticipating the delivery of your catalog of possibilities and beliefs.

Expect to receive powerful visions of what you have the power to manifest.

Once your catalog has arrived, peruse it and start making a list of the possible projects inviting themselves into your life.

Enjoy the process of attracting your possibilities as you watch them present themselves to you.

Your Map to "I'll Attract My Catalog, Review My Options, and Decide What I Want"

Know that you can create the results you desire using this formula.

Develop an attitude of complete responsibility for your life.

Decide exactly what you want.

Be sure you have the interest and belief that you can have what you want. Then you will be prepared to put your goals in writing and develop the capacity to visualize the result and create a schedule for what you need to do.

Your Map to "I'll Develop Interest and Belief"

Develop and cultivate genuine interest in manifesting the things you want that appear in your catalog of possibilities.

Make sure you really believe these things can by yours and that you can accomplish whatever you set your mind and talents to creating.

Be prepared to do the work that will need to be done to stick to your commitment and to set goals that you will accomplish.

Your Map to "I'll Create My Goals and Put Them in Writing"

Put your goals in writing, and develop the capacity to visualize your results.
Add animation to your goals, giving them movement and life.
Create a schedule for what you need to do.
Know the practical steps you'll need to take to get to your desire results.
Be prepared to do the work and enjoy the results.

Your Map to "I'll Go Fast Like a Tortoise"

Have your goals in writing.
Give yourself plenty of time to accomplish the work that needs to be done.
Know that, to have quality results, you'll have to invest quality time and that the process is like planting seeds and should be enjoyed.
Watch your efforts grow like seeds.
Enjoy feeling the changes and the increase of the good that you experience.
Keep moving slowly but surely toward your goal.

Your Map to "I'll Become Magnetic"

See yourself as a magnet. Develop the belief that you draw to you exactly what you need when you need it.
Always be on the lookout for inspiration that will nudge you toward your success.

Act on the inspiration you attract. Taking action will guarantee more guidance in the future.

Your Map to "I'll Do the Work, Let Go of the Experience, and Keep the Lesson"

Take responsibility for your thinking and your memory. See the experiences you've had as opportunities for learning. Remember what you've learned. Forget the details of how you got here.

Avoid shoulding. Change "I should" to "I choose to _____."

See yourself as the creator of our own museum. Display your collection of treasures that you collected on your journey.

Your Map to "I'll Celebrate"

Put a cherry on top of your goal by knowing that the effort you put into it deserves recognition. Vividly visualize yourself as a success, worthy of celebrating.

See the celebration. Imagine the location and the guest list, and see yourself thanking all those who helped and supported you along the way.

Vividly see yourself returning to what was your old world with all the loot you gathered on your journey: higher esteem, deeper faith in yourself and your abilities, a new strong and successful presence, and a spirited sense of going back for more.

About the Author

ARTHUR Hammons is a member of the National Speakers Association. He is a veteran of inspiring and helping people discover and build the life they want. His keynote presentation and book, *Yes! You Can Do This!*, speak to the heart of addressing how to set and reach goals.

As chief executive officer and founder of Christ Church Unity of El Cajon, California, where he served for 38 years, he has officiated at more than 4,000 weddings and 1,500 funerals and memorial services. He hosted the popular TV program *There Is a Way* for 10 years to an audience of over 1,000,000 viewers each week. He co-authored the book *Out of Your Mind*.

Arthur stimulates thinking, dreaming, and accomplishing in the people he speaks to, as well as gives them a sense of personal empowerment and the tools to craft a plan for creating health, wealth, better relationships, and productiveness. His presentations are tailored to issues of greatest concern, including strategies for developing a system for staying focused and performing at one's best daily. Arthur's one-of-a-kind philosophy has the right combination of wisdom, insight, ideas, and passion that are practical and can be implemented immediately. Arthur provides people with what they need to know about identifying their goals and desires, and bringing them to accomplishment.

Arthur lives in La Jolla, California, with his wife, Dr. Virginia Foster. He enjoys running half-marathons, riding his horse, painting, and creating with stained glass.

For further information about Arthur's books and presentations, contact him:

Phone: (619) 851–0203
E-mail: Garthurhammons@aol.com
Web: www.ArthurHammons.com